D1242653

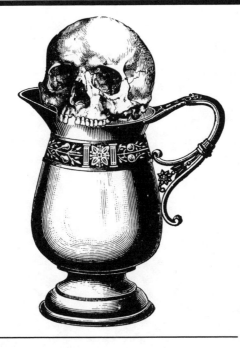

Poison
in the Pot
The Legacy of Lead

Richard P. Wedeen, M.D., F.A.C.P.

Southern Illinois University Press

Carbondale and Edwardsville

Library of Congress Cataloging in Publication Data

Wedeen, Richard P., 1934–
Poison in the pot: the legacy of lead.

Bibliography: p.
Includes index.
1. Nephritis, Interstitial—Etiology.   2. Lead-poisoning.
3. Occupational diseases.   I. Title. [DNLM:
1. Lead poisoning—History.   2. Kidney diseases—
Etiology.   3. Gout—Etiology.   4. Gout—History.
5. Lead poisoning—Complications.   6. Kidney diseases—
History. QV 292 W389p]
RC918.N37W43   1984   616.6'12   84-2296
ISBN 0-8093-1156-9

Printed in the United States of America

Edited by Stephen W. Smith

Designed by Rich Hendel

Production supervised by Kathleen Giencke

87 86 85 84   4 3 2 1

Contents

Figures

Preface

Medical research on the effect of lead has lured me into the realm of medical history. It seems strangely anachronistic to approach modern medical science with historical tales, looking backward as well as forward. Homage to classical authority became unfashionable in the eighteenth century, but modern scientific medicine also has its revered authorities whose conventional wisdom tenaciously resists change. It is, therefore, not inappropriate to argue from arcane texts that modern medicine may have forgotten criticial insights about the dangers of lead. History, indeed, repeats itself in the resistance of practitioners to unconventional concepts and the resultant cost to human health.

In contrast to the marshaling of data appropriate to scientific arguments, I will present lead poisoning and gout in their historical framework, as often as possible in the writers' own words. I have relied on direct quotation to let authors speak for themselves, but review the subject with the unabashed bias of a participant in the controversy. The foibles of past and present are confronted in the belief that ideas may be explained, but not excused, by the societal framework in which they are created. To be relevant to the present, contemporary criteria of medical reality are applied equally. As an investigator freed, for the moment, of the uniform, dry, and sometimes neutered style obligatory in medical journals, I avoid equivocation. Were I to reply to the historian's criticism, I might let John Donne plead for me (196):

> For God's sake hold your tongue, and let me love,
>   Or chide my palsy, or my gout.
> My five gray hairs, or ruined fortune flout,
>   . . . what you will, approve,
> So you will let me love.

(p. 473)

To those who mourn the passing of the general practitioner, medical history seen through a single syndrome may seem symptomatic of over-specialization. On the other hand, a grasp of specific details may provide insight unavailable to the generalist. A close examination of the trees need not obscure the forest but may, in fact, reveal its timber far more vividly than the grand perspective.

Physicians have not been alone in their attempts to grapple with the insidious scourge of lead. A persistent intermingling of lead in wine and rum placed this metal at the core of social history. Poets and philosophers, preachers and satirists have created a lore about wine and gout which is an integral part of the story. Their frustrations and delights not infrequently reflect the impact of medicine on the human condition. This plumbing of the depths of medical history is therefore undertaken in the hope that the interplay between scholars and quacks, scientists and merchants, pleasure and suffering is worth retelling. The uneasy flow of knowledge has an eloquence of its own from which, perhaps, some lessons can be relearned.

In the *Anatomy of Melancholy*, Robert Burton could not "omit those two main plagues and common dotages of human kind, Wine and Women, which have infatuated and besotted Myriads of people" (106, p. 72). Yet, he assures us, "to such as are cold, or sluggish melancholy, a cup of Wine is good Physic" (p. 42).

Both earlier and later physicians have agreed with Burton. Their ambivalence toward wine has many sources. Sometimes by design, sometimes by accident, alcoholic drinks have been contaminated with lead through the ages. The result has been repeated epidemics of gout, colic, palsy, and worse. Not all the mysteries of lead have yet been solved, and some that were solved have, from time to time, been forgotten.

It is believed that there are at least 850,000 lead workers in the United States, and that a million Americans suffer from gout. If this reexamination of history leads to treatment and prevention of disease in a fraction of this population, then these tales can perhaps be of service as well as interest. Lead nephropathy offers a unique opportunity to physicians, because the cause can not only be determined, but the disease can be prevented and sometimes reversed. In the majority of chronic renal diseases not even the etiology can be ascertained with confidence.

I AM INDEBTED TO those whose assistance and encouragement have made this endeavor delightful: L. Fred Ayvazian, M.D., William Ober, M.D., Marshall Clemens, Dorothy Hanks, William Helfand, and Michael Sollenberger. I am also grateful to my partners in ongoing research on lead and the kidney: Vecihi Batuman, M.D., Claffertene Cheeks, Keith Jones, Ph.D., Hobart Kraner, Ph.D., Elaine Landy, R.N., John Maesaka, M.D., and Michael Nystrom.

Prologue

Every clinical intervention carries with it the essence of the scientific method. Uncontrollable variables, however, undermine generalizations from a single diagnostic or therapeutic maneuver. More extended trials are called for with precisely defined controls. Thus, clinical experience generates testable hypotheses and "an interesting case" can mold a medical career. It was just such a case that enticed me into studies of the renal consequences of lead, lead nephropathy. A recurring pattern of medical misunderstandings soon became evident. Tales both amusing and amazing emerged on all sides, confined to no single place or time. The dilemmas of the present reiterated dilemmas of the past. Colic followed by palsy, and gout are distinctive and protracted consequences of lead poisoning; they can be identified as such in even the most ancient descriptions. The roots of present controversies were thus readily traced to the past. The possibility that the impact of lead on health in the past could be proved by contemporary methods was irresistible. The conviction that lead nephropathy had been largely overlooked by modern physicians opened a morass of questions that led me into the realm of medical history.

Until recently, textbooks and governmental guidelines alike claimed that kidney disease due to occupational lead exposure rarely occurred in the United States because of this country's advanced industrial-health practices (755). It was generally agreed that lead intoxication was seen chiefly in the industrialized nations of Europe where less effective occupational health standards prevailed. Lead nephropathy was relegated to the distant past and to the underdeveloped countries of the world. Kidney damage was believed to occur only when the blood lead was markedly elevated (819). Moreover, the notion that interstitial disease of the kidneys was due to undetected bacterial invasion (pyelonephritis) inhibited attempts to identify other specific causes of nonglomerular kidney disease. Such authoritative dicta diverted American physicians from making the diagnosis of occupational lead nephropathy.

In this context, in 1971 I saw in consultation a young man who had been hospitalized with abdominal pain and anemia. This was his sixth hospital admission for similar complaints over two years. With each hospitalization a different diagnosis had been made: hepatitis, ulcer, gastritis, gall bladder, virus, and neurosis. His gall bladder had been removed with subsequent relief of the pain. In fact, any in-hospital treatment seemed to relieve the excruciating abdominal cramps, but a month or two after returning to work his pains recurred.

For five years he had manufactured solder to be used for electrical connections. He prepared solder creams by converting molten lead into powder in a small unventilated room. One physician, suspecting lead poisoning, had drawn blood for measurement of lead. But the patient's blood level was reported to be within what was then an "acceptable" range: less than 80 μg of lead per 100 ml. The diagnosis of lead poisoning could not be established.

Despite the paucity of information on lead and the kidney, our patient's complaints demanded attention. Methodology to prove the diagnosis of asymptomatic lead poisoning could not be found in the federal guidelines but had to be sought elsewhere. To the traditional symptoms of colic followed by the palsy, modern biochemists had added sophisticated laboratory tests of blood and urine. Anemia and immature red blood cells had been associated with plumbism in the nineteenth century. The defects in red cell production induced by lead could now be detected by exquisitely sensitive tests of heme synthesis. Highly accurate measurements of the blood lead concentration were also available. Blood lead had become the canon of laboratory diagnosis, a status that was to falter during the period of these investigations.

The available evidence suggested that neither the classical symptoms nor current biochemical tests would suffice to detect dangerous lead stores accumulated slowly over many years. Tests of urine and blood had found favor because of convenience, the accessibility of both methodology and the body fluids. But lead differs from most environmental toxins in that once it enters the body it is stored in the bones. Over 95 percent of the body lead is retained in bone where it persists for many years. The biological half life of bone lead is estimated to be several decades. This lead storage provides the potential for both delayed toxicity and diagnostic assessment. I chose, therefore, to rely upon a rather cumbersome diagnostic procedure validated for lead nephropathy in Australia a decade earlier, the EDTA lead-mobilization test.

The EDTA test requires two injections and the formidable task of collecting accurate twenty-four-hour urine specimens. The injections are anathema to patients while the urine collections become a logistical nightmare when large numbers of patients are studied. Despite the inconvenience, the EDTA lead-mobilization test promised identification of individuals at high risk for lead nephropathy, including those who had never had colic or neurologic symptoms and in whom abnormalities of blood or urine had never been recorded. In these individuals, lead poisoning would have gone unrecognized by patient and physician alike. Traditional diagnostic techniques were unreliable for the detection of long-term, low-level lead exposure in the past.

Using the EDTA lead-mobilization test, I demonstrated that lead poisoning was the most likely cause of the abdominal pain and anemia in our patient. Evidence of mild kidney disease was even more difficult to interpret since American authorities doubted the existence of occupational lead nephropathy.

Because our conclusions conflicted with prevailing opinion, we carefully measured the patient's kidney function and found it to be reduced by 40 percent. His kidney biopsy showed nonspecific interstitial nephritis. A course of deleading by EDTA therapy was begun. From time to time we reestimated his body lead stores and renal function. These serial studies showed that as the lead was removed, his kidney function progressively improved. The effectiveness of the specific treatment provided compelling confirmation of the diagnosis of lead nephropathy (794).

Having identified one case of occupational lead nephropathy despite claims in the literature that the entity did not exist, my colleagues and I decided to look for additional cases. The force of economic pressure immediately became apparent. None of our patient's co-workers agreed to be examined, nor would they sign a request for a plant inspection by the Occupational Safety and Health Administration (OSHA). The local union representatives refused to discuss the matter. We were warned against pressing a confrontation.

Aid in finding workers at risk for lead nephropathy finally came from Dr. Irving Selikoff at the Mt. Sinai Medical School. Dr. Selikoff had gained international recognition for revealing the full impact of asbestos on workers in that industry. His laboratory, consequently, had considerable leverage in occupation health circles. Drs. Susan Daum and Ruth Lilis of his department played a key role in arranging to have me meet our patient's employers. I recounted the findings and their implications to the corporation's representatives. There was a lively interest in the issues raised. The employers thanked us for the information, expressed interest in pursuing the problem of lead exposure in their plant, but advised me explicitly, "Don't call us, we will call you."

With the guidance of the Mt. Sinai staff, I eventually found a union local near my research laboratory in Jersey City, that was interested in finding out if its members were lead-poisoned. The plant was under threat of closure, and the employees believed they were about to be laid off.

During the next year, we examined thirty men for excessive lead stores. Among eight with abnormal amounts of lead in their bodies, four were found to have hitherto unsuspected renal disease for which no other explanation could be found. Suddenly, lead nephropathy did not appear to be at all rare in American industry.

A preliminary report of our data entitled, "Blood Lead—An Inadequate Measure Of Occupational Exposure" (768), brought refutation from industry (395) and government alike. Letters protesting our conclusions were published in the *Journal of Occupational Medicine* (151, 457). Six months later, when our detailed findings appeared, the outrage was less articulate. I did, however, receive a personal letter from the Department of Occupational Health of a prominent university. Rather pleased at the interest shown in our work, I answered the criticism in a detailed three-page response, affirming the conclusion that our four patients did, indeed, have occupational lead nephropathy. To my amazement, six months later I received a galley proof of this correspondence from the *American Journal of Medicine*.

Unknown to me, the *Journal* had initiated a policy of printing "Letters to the Editor." More surprising still was the fact that my academic colleague had, without my knowledge, submitted our correspondence for publication. My correspondent, it developed, was a consultant to the lead industry in addition to being a member of the university's faculty. I revised the letter to include documentation of his role as an industry spokesman and returned it to the editor of the *Ameican Journal of Medicine* (786).

The controversy generated by these studies took place in an arena that was new to me. My previous research had been in basic cell biology with little socioeconomic impact. Now I was asked to testify before a Senate oversight hearing and a Department of Labor regulatory meeting. Whenever I presented our findings, industry spokesmen issued volumes denying their significance. Despite such protests and the refusal of the National Institute of Occupational Safety and Health to fund our research, our data were in great demand by other government agencies. The Environmental Protection Agency, The National Institute of Environmental Safety and Health, The Occupational Safety and Health Administration clamored for our report even before it was ready for publication.

It was clear that the standard technique for detecting excessive lead absorption—determination of the blood lead concentration—was grossly inadequate to identify workers at risk for occupational lead nephropathy. The insensitivity of the blood lead to the level of exposure had been one of the better kept secrets of the lead industry for fifty years (338). Because many of the men we studied had terminated their lead exposure months earlier, the EDTA lead-mobilization test was required to find those with excessive body lead stores. Over five years, twenty-one cases of unsuspected renal disease among lead workers were discovered. In fifteen, no other cause of renal disease could be found, and in 4, the lead nephropathy was reversed by long-term chelation therapy (794). The existence of renal disease in asymptomatic lead workers was soon confirmed by others (29, 101, 383, 466–70, 760). The inadequacy of the blood lead for detection of patients with excessive absorption of lead in the past was also noted by others (14, 361). Furthermore, the widely held belief that chelation therapy with $CaNa_2EDTA$ is contraindicated in the presence of renal failure was contraverted by the improvement in renal function in treated patients (198). Further experience indicated that the EDTA lead-mobilization test was not nephrotoxic even in the presence of preexisting renal disease (792).

The "interesting case" embroiled me in a range of controversies that had long surrounded lead poisoning. After removing the excessive lead stores with EDTA therapy, the patient's renal function returned to normal. This encouraging result was, however, negated five years later when he developed gout, hypertension, and a return of his renal failure. The relationship of gout, hypertension, and renal disease to each other as well as to lead poisoning had provoked volatile debate among physicians for a century. Controversy over the origin of gout was, itself, a venerable tradition in medicine. Saturnine gout, well described in the eighteenth century, was virtually unknown to medical students of the 1980s. But these questions remained for future exploration. For the moment, my concern was to establish the existence of occupational lead nephropathy.

In 1978, OSHA released new regulations for lead exposure in the workplace. In relation to lead-induced kidney disease this "Occupational Exposure to Lead Final Standard" states (757):

One of the most important contributions to the understanding of adverse health effects associated with exposure to inorganic lead was the elucidation of evidence on kidney disease during the hearings. It is apparent that kidney disease from exposure to lead is far more prevalent than previously believed. In the past, the number of lead workers with kidney disease in the United States was thought to be negligible, but the record indicates that a substantial number of workers may be afflicted with this disease. Wedeen, a nephrologist (kidney specialist), who testified at the hearings for OSHA stated that a minimal estimate of the incidence of this disease (nephropathy) would be 10 percent of lead workers. According to this estimate, "there may be 100,000 cases of preventable renal disease in this country. . . . If only 10 percent of these hundred thousand workers came to chronic hemodialysis (kidney machines) the cost to Medicare alone would be about 200 million dollars per year" (p. 52958).

The "Final Standard" presented a detailed analysis of the conclusions from our preliminary studies.

OSHA agrees with the conclusions of Wedeen: "By the time lead nephropathy can be detected by usual clinical procedures, enormous and irreparable damage has been sustained. The lead standard must be directed towards limiting exposure so that occupational lead nephropathy does not occur," since in this situation "progression to death or dialysis is likely." The record indicates that blood lead is an inadequate indicator of kidney disease development, since rather than being a complete measure of body burden, it is merely a measure of absorption when sampled close to the time of exposure. Given these conclusions, OSHA must approach the prevention of kidney disease by recognizing the limited usefulness of certain biological parameters. Therefore, OSHA believes any standard established for lead must provide some margin of safety.

The lead standard must therefore be directed towards limiting exposure so that occupational lead nephropathy is prevented. The Agency agrees with the views of Wedeen: "Lead nephropathy is important because the worker has lost the functional reserve, the safety provided by two normal kidneys. If one kidney becomes damaged, the normal person has another to rely upon. The lead worker with 50 percent loss of kidney function has no such security. Future loss of kidney function will normally occur with increasing age, and may be accelerated by hypertension or infection. The usual life processes will bring the lead worker to the point of uremia, while the normal individual still has considerable renal functional reserve. Loss of a kidney is therefore more serious than loss of an arm, for example. Loss of an arm leads to obvious limitations in activity. Loss of a kidney or an equivalent loss of kidney function means the lead worker's ability to survive the biologic events of life is severely reduced."

And OSHA agrees with Dr. Richard Wedeen, that "40 μg/100 is the upper acceptable limit" (p. 52959).

In preparing the "Final Standard" a new philosophy was formulated concerning the responsibility of government in protecting the health of industrial workers. Rather than awaiting the onset of clinical symptoms. OSHA had accepted responsibility for preventing organ damage. The crucial concept is that subtle, but measurable, biologic derangements are considered evidence of "materially impaired health" even when detected only in the laboratory. The worker, then, does not have to be symptomatic to be recognized as ill: the so-called "preclinical" or "subclinical" effects of lead must also be prevented. Occupational health specialists are more accustomed to cancer incidence data than to physiologic estimates of kidney function. But evidence that lead causes renal cancer in man (as it does in rodents) is virtually nonexistent (28). The regulatory bodies were therefore forced to come to terms with the more abstract measurements of preclinical organ dysfunction in the blood, nervous system, and the kidneys. Impairment of the enzymes responsible for synthesis of hemoglobin has been demonstrated at blood lead levels as low as 18 μg/dl (605). Laboratory evidence of lead-induced defects in heme synthesis is now considered indicative of organ damage. Public pressure to reduce the "acceptable" blood level towards 18 μg/dl may soon prove irresistible.

The potential financial impact of the new federal regulations did not escape the attention of industry. The lead companies sued. On June 29, 1981, the United States Supreme Court denied the industry's claims: the Court upheld the obligation of OSHA to protect industrial workers without first providing proof of "cost-effectiveness." Defeat in court shifted the lead industry's attacks directly to the regulatory agencies themselves. The dismantling of NIOSH, OSHA, and the EPA became the most effective route for delaying implementation of the "Final Standard."

With the publication of the "Final Standard," American medical opinion on lead nephropathy reverted to that of the nineteenth century. Occupational lead nephropathy once again received official recognition (29). Such turnabouts do not come easily but are by no means unheard of in medicine. Unconventional ideas have never been eagerly received by physicians. Orthodoxy is impressed upon the biomedical community by the presence of "experts" on research grant and editorial review panels. Reviewers resist new ideas for three reasons: 1) If the expert agrees, he would have performed the studies himself. 2) If he disagrees, his own theories are, in all likelihood, in jeopardy. 3) Defects tend to be more glaring to the reviewer in work which refutes his own point of view than in work which supports him. Expertise itself introduces conservatism if not bias. An old-boy network exists wherein reviewers are more likely to trust the assertions of investigators with whom they share academic experience and insight. The proponents of conventional work are supported, while delays in funding or publication of unorthodox ideas may cause unconventional research to perish. In the field of environmental toxicology, unadvertised financial support of selected experts by the lead industry, both directly and indirectly, makes it particularly difficult to gain acceptance of new ideas which might increase manufacturing costs.

Conventionality in research, however, is not entirely useless. Maverick ideas can only be incorporated into a structure of existing knowledge. Deviations from the norm are properly viewed with suspicion. Science requires consistency: a cautious and conservative safeguard against blunder. New concepts, like radical politics, meet resistance until internalized by the establishment.

The major difference in the adoption of unconventional ideas in the twentieth, as compared to the sixteenth century, is the speed of change. Shifts in thinking occur in decades rather than centuries, as conceptualization forever chases technology. Methodologic advances sire new experimental generations about every ten years: roughly the span required for the limitations of current techniques to be appreciated. Transitions in thinking are rarely abrupt. Conformity is quickly reestablished, as last year's renegade hypothesis is adapted and adopted, fashioned into the new conventionality. Conceptual evolution has been telescoped from centuries to decades, but experimental surprises remain inherently unwelcome.

Resistance to change is easily masked by scientific skepticism, which may serve as a convenient guise for obstructionism. But new ideas and irrepressible questions disrupt complacency. The evolution of clinical concepts of lead poisoning and lead-induced gout (saturnine gout) have proven too provocative to ignore. While lead has been found to be responsible for ever more subtle injuries to man, gout has evolved into an ever more benign disease. The once virulent gout has been quieted; only renal disease and hypertension remain as its feared complications. These changing faces of disease might merely reflect changing medical fashions; physicians' conceptions rather than the diseases may have changed. Older concepts of gout may simply have been medical fantasies derived from humoral doctrine appropriately abandoned along with outdated theories. On the other hand, the evolution of medical concepts of gout may represent the changing frequency of encounters with a surreptitious saturnine malady. The variable incidence of unrecognized lead poisoning might account for the change in the clinical syndrome.

Knowledge of the impact of lead on health has evolved over two thousand years and medical resistance to changing concepts of its toxicity has been as constant as the disease itself. Lulled by familiarity, physicians and public alike are not easily aroused by claims of new dangers from this venerable poison.

Vested interests are superimposed on medical complacency. The enormous value of lead to society adds another dimension to the usual resistance to change. Economic and professional bias have bolstered conservative views throughout history while fear of the unfamiliar excites far more attention than fear of the commonplace. But, like science itself, human self-interest shows signs of being self-correcting. The history of industrial health practices suggests that protection of man from man-made hazards is not only possible but, in the long run, likely to prevail.

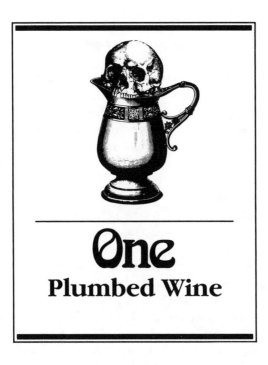

One
Plumbed Wine

The Historical Perspective

Ecologic hazard as a by-product of technologic progress is not unique to modern civilization. Mankind's use of lead began over eight millennia ago, probably in the region of the Aegean Sea. An ordinary campfire achieves temperatures sufficient to smelt lead from galena, an abundant ore containing lead sulfide. Lead beads dating from 6500 B.C. have been found at Catal Huyuk in Asia Minor (281) and a lead statue believed to date from 3800 B.C. was found in the temple of Osiris in Abydos, Egypt. Essential to the extraction of iron from crude ore, lead smelting was the harbinger of the Iron Age (800).

The economic strength of Athens was founded on lead. Products of the Attic mines have been identified in the royal tombs of Crete, Mycenae, and Egypt. It has been suggested that it was this trade with Crete that brought Theseus to visit King Minos in the Bronze Age (282). Theseus' confrontation with the Minotaur might thus be a mythological metaphor for more mundane commercial adventures. The ancient mines of Thorikon are still to be found on a brush-covered hill overlooking the Aegean.

Just four kilometers from the active port of Lavrion, nestled within one hundred yards of a classic Greek amphitheater is the small but carefully chiseled entrance to the subterranean chamber. Nearby, the ruins of metallurgical shops have been unearthed by archeologists. On an adjacent hill, modern smelters, complete with contemporary slag heaps, are alive with activity. Smog hugs the shallow valley spanning six thousand years of economic progress. Lead ores were long ago exhausted from the Attic Peninsula. Now, freighters bring galena from Egypt, reversing the trade lanes plied by the ancient Greeks.

By 1200 B.C., the Romans were skillful in the use of metals for the enrichment of everyday life (6, 554). Their utensils and armaments exploited the metallurgists' skills. As luxury increased with empire, the villas of ancient Rome were adorned with wall to wall mosaics and equipped with lead plumbing. Murals depicting the *dolce vita* of the patricians were painted with lead pigments: vivid white and Pompeian red. The women of Rome adorned themselves with lead pigments, the manufacture of which had been described by Theophrastus in ancient Greece but undoubtedly antedates written history (746).

The Romans found that wine served in lead vessels was sweeter and kept fresh longer. Alerted to the danger of drinking water carried in lead pipes by Vitruvius and Galen (145), they were apparently unaware of the dangers of lead added to the fruit of the vine. Cato, Pliny, and Columella each advised that the juice of the grapes be boiled in lead vessels to enhance flavor and prevent undue fermentation (554, 555, 730), a practice pursued by vintners well into the nineteenth century (223).

As opulence increased, liberated Roman women shared the wine. Poisoned by the lead in their food, kitchenware, and cosmetics, they suffered not only abdominal pains, paralysis of peripheral nerves, and encephalopathy but also infertility. It has been hypothesized that this infertility contributed to the fall of Rome. "Lead poisoning," wrote Gilfillan, "of the wives and mistresses of upper class Romans occurred chiefly through their diet, after the introduction of Greek cookery around 150 B.C. and the relaxation of the old rule against wives drinking wine. The most significant sources of lead were wine, grape syrup, and preserved fruit. The Roman free poor and the slaves had much less lead in their diet" (306, p. 54).

According to this hypothesis, lead-laden repasts were luxuries for the masters who indulged themselves nearly to extinction. The food and drink of the rich were well preserved. Fermentation was inhibited by generous admixing with lead salts extracted by organic acids and slow cooking. Mulled wine, simmered in lead kettles, was a favorite in the taverns of Pompeii (554). Although the deleterious effects were sometimes recognized in occupational exposure, the slower, more subtle poisoning from wine was difficult to pinpoint. Plumbism was easily confused with alcoholism, as it is still today. The resulting sterility and high rate of miscarriage was, however, of considerable concern to the aristocracy of Rome. "The Romans recognized what was happening," Gilfillan concludes. "The bachelor, Horace, persuaded Augustus, who had only a daughter, to pass laws penalizing aristocratic bachelors, and granting special privileges, the *Jus trium liberorum*, to the fathers of 3 or more children" (p. 57). But the attempt to increase the progeny of the ruling class was to no avail. The strength of the aristocracy was sapped while their slaves, denied the culinary poison, increased in numbers and eventually displaced the declining patricians. The decrease in birth rate due to lead may have had a devastating impact on successive generations. Although the cause of infertility was not recognized, the more worldly Roman ladies regarded preparations of lead applied to the cervix as an effective means of contraception, an old wives' tale circulated by Aristotle (554).

While Gilfillan's provocative thesis has been criticized for having more literary than scientific merit, this objection may well be resolved in the future by bone lead measurements in archeological specimens. When such studies have been attempted in the past, the social status of the exhumed Romans was not accurately known. The bones of slave-owners in seventeenth-century Virginia, however, have been shown to contain distinctly toxic levels of lead while their slaves were spared this burden of opulence (23).

While the deliberate use of lead in wine spread with Roman civilization, the origin of knowledge of its sweetening and preserving effects on fermented liquors is lost in history (258, 554). Lead mining and smelting were widely practiced in the Bronze Age. In northern China, from 2000 to 900 B.C., cast bronze vessels contained progressively increasing quantities of lead (472). These magnificent objects sometimes contained up to 98 percent of the plentiful heavy metal. If Chinese custom condoned imbibing as well as libations, it is likely that ancient eastern rituals had painful consequences.

Both Hippocrates and Galen commented on the dangers of metallurgical occupations. Slaves forced to labor in the silver mines of ancient Greece rarely survived over five years. If they outlived brutality, they succumbed to lead poisoning. Silver was extracted from lead ores at least as early as 2500 B.C. on Siphnos in the Cyclades (770). By the time of the

Roman Empire the more malleable by-product was obtained in a thousandfold greater quantities than silver (590). Roman silver mining resulted in a massive increase in the use of lead, which was exceeded, in terms of environmental pollution, only during the industrial revolution (681).

In 200 B.C. Nikander of Colophon, hereditary priest of Apollo, poet-philosopher, and physician, recorded some of the effects of lead poisoning.

> But may the hateful, painful litharge
>   be unknown to you,
> If oppression rages in your belly,
>   and all around your middle,
> Pent up in your howling bowels
>   winds roar,
> The sort which cause deadly disturbances
>   of the bowels, which,
> Attacking with pains unexpected,
>   overpower mankind.
> The flood of urine does not stop it,
>   but all around
> The limbs are swollen and inflamed,
> And, no less, the skin's color
>   is that of lead.

In the first century of the Christian era, Nikander's knowledge of lead poisoning was reiterated by Dioscorides and known to Pliny the Elder, who advised the use of animal bladders as face masks to protect workmen from the dust of red lead (607). Paul of Aegina recounted Dioscorides' description of lead colic, anemia, and renal disease in the seventh century (5).

> Litharge [lead oxide], when drunk brings on heaviness of the stomach and bowels, with intense tormina; sometimes by its weight it wounds the intestines, occasions retention of urine and swelling of the body, which becomes of a leaden hue, and assumes an unseemly appearance. . . . When a person has drunk the shavings of lead or its soil, he experiences the same symptoms as those from litharge, and is to be treated in the same manner (p. 237).

Writing of "paralysis supervening upon colic disease," Paul of Aegina also described the combination of colic with neurologic symptoms, without, however, realizing the cause. Paul was aware of this problem in ancient Rome.

> I am of the opinion that the colic affection which now prevails is occasioned by such humours: the disease having taken its rise in the country of Italy, but raging also in many other regions of the Roman empire, like a pestilential contagion, which in many cases terminates in epilepsy, but in others in paralysis of the extremities, while the sensibility of them is preserved, and sometimes both these affections attacking together. And of those who fell into epilepsy the greater number died: but of the paralytics the most recovered, as their complaint proved a critical metastasis of the cause of the disorder (p. 534).

From the second to the sixteenth centuries original medical observations virtually vanished in Europe. Learning was replaced by stultifying repetition of classical authority. Chemistry was relegated to the shadowy alchemists whose empirical knowledge of alloys formed the foundation of later science.

During the Dark Ages, Arabian physicians became the repository for Greek and Roman medical knowledge as Europe cowered before God and Church. Avicenna recalled the Roman experience when writing of "well water and water conveyed along aqueducts." "Of such waters," the Islamic master observed, "those which are conveyed by leaden pipes are more harmful, because they acquire certain properties of the lead, and this makes them liable to bring on a certain form of dysentery [colic]" (25, p. 225). Avicenna was also cognizant of the dire consequences of medicinal lead (33). In 1198, Maimonides, the Jewish physician who fled to Egypt in order to pursue his studies, counted "martak (plumbum oxydatum) [and] saccharum saturni (lithargyros)" (p. 59) first among the deadly mineral poisons (505). Charlemagne is reputed to have outlawed the adulteration of wine with lead in 802 (223).

Medicine languished in Europe, but artisans remembered some of the lessons of the ancient physicians. In an admirable treatise "On Divers Arts" published at the beginning of the twelfth century, Theophilus cautioned metalworkers to remove the lead from brass to avoid "the various accidents that are wont to happen to men when they are gilding" (p. 139) in the presence of lead (745).

While the consequences of lead poisoning were but vaguely perceived, the differential diagnosis of colic was totally obscure. There was no way to distinguish dysentery from obstructed bowel or lead colic. In the most popular of early printed texts, colic was equated with retained flatus, the venting of which was strongly advised (356).

Great harmes have growne, & maladies exceeding,
By keeping in a little blast of wind:
So Cramps & Dropsies, Collickes haue
   their breeding,
And Mazed Braines for Want of vent behind:

(p. 79)

This warning from the English version of the *School of Salerno* had been accompanied by a very explicit illustration from an earlier Latin publication of the same lore (fig. 1). The colic accompanied by a palsy was not perceived as distinctive in Renaissance Europe. That lead poisoning was, nevertheless, commonplace is evident from recurring laws requiring the elimination of lead from alcoholic beverages (33, 98, 223, 730).

With the resurgence of secular learning many of the lessons of the past had to be rediscovered. Thirteenth-century Latin translations of Islamic scholars such as Jabir ibn Hayyan of the eighth century (known as Geber in medieval Europe), Rhazes of the ninth and Avicenna of the tenth century, transmitted considerable metallurgical sophistication to fifteenth-century Europe. In 1473, Ulrich Ellenbog wrote perhaps the first treatise on occupational health (224, 225), *On The Poisonous Evil Vapours and Fumes of Metals such as Silver, Quicksilver, Lead and Others*. In his advice to "the nobel craft of goldsmiths and other workers," Ellenbog warned against the fumes of metals. "Lead is a cold poison," he explained, "for it maketh heaviness and tightness of the chest, burdeneth the limbs and ofttimes lameth them as often one seeth in foundries where men do work with large masses and the vital inward members become burdened therefrom" (225, p. 271). Recognizing that avoiding the noxious vapors was not always feasible, he advised that musk be kept nearby. Its vapors would counteract the "coldness" of the lead. Further protection could be obtained by the workman's holding in his mouth a variety of substances including juniper berries, rue, dittany, or emeralds. This brief treatise published in 1524 was a forerunner of the first comprehensive work on the refining of metals published by Georgius Agricola in 1555, *De Re Metallica* (6).

Woodcuts accompanying Agricola's text illustrated the smelting process. They show that laborers were heavily exposed to the fumes of lead

DE FLATVS VENTRIS
retentione. CAP. IILI.

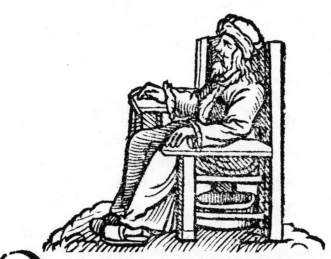

Q Vatuor ex uento ueniunt in uen
tre retento:
Spafmus, hydrops, colica , & uertigo
quatuor ifta.

*1. The venting of flatus as depicted in a 1551 edition of the health wisdom of
the* School of Salerno *(174).*

even when the work was performed in the open (fig. 2). Although himself
a physician, Agricola did not describe lead colic, which must have been
prevalent under these conditions. However, in a text on minerals published in 1546, he counseled that ingestion of lead dissolved in vinegar
could be fatal (7).

Following the intimidation of the Middle Ages, the distillation of information was a slow and uncertain process in which lingering mysticism
confounded observation. By the end of the sixteenth century, only a few
scholars were privy to the symptoms of lead poisoning. Jean Fernel knew
of the dangers of medicinal lead, but we have from George Baker the following passage (33):

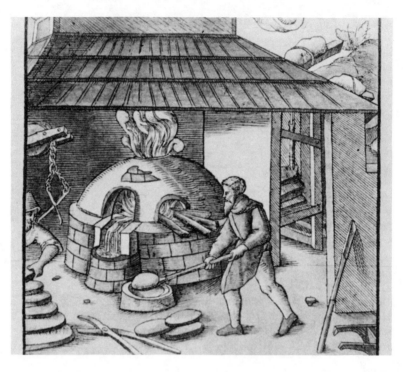

2. Lead is a major by-product in the extraction of silver. From De Re Metallica *by Georgius Agricola, first published in 1555 (6).*

It seems wonderful to find, how very little, physicians, even of the first reputation, formerly knew of the deleterious qualities of lead. Fernelius who published his *Universa Medicina* in the year 1592, although, in his seventh chapter *de lues venerae curatione*, he describes most terrible effects of the powder of lead, given, in the quantity of a pound and half, in the space of fifteen days, to his friend, as a remedy against the gout; (which effects he attributes to the hidden and inexplicable malignity of that metal; and concludes from that case, that lead ought never to be taken into the body) in the very same page, when he describes the true colic of Poitou, in the case of a painter of Anjou, in the year 1557, plainly shews, that neither he, nor any of the other physicians concerned, understood the true cause of the disease (p. 342).

While traditional humoral doctrine could accommodate a plethora of natural and supernatural phenomena, such dogma obscured causal relationships. Even when colic followed by the palsy reached epidemic proportions, the toxic etiology went unrecognized. But in a quixotic universe governed by unfathomable forces, such epidemics served to focus attention, a first step toward understanding.

Colic of Poitou

In 1639, François Citois described a devastating epidemic of colic in the town of Potiers, in the wine district of Poitou, which he called "dolor colica Pictonum" (146) but which was commonly referred to as the "colic of Poitou." In retrospect, the symptoms were unquestionably due to lead poisoning.

Citois attributed the colic of Poitou to permutations of astrological and natural factors including the stars, the air, the climate, food, acrid acid, and urine. The allusion to astrological signs stemmed from a supernovae, described by Tycho Brahe, which appeared in the heavens at the time (223). Citois believed that the bilious humor was the direct cause of the pain and he incidentally confused lead, ureteral, and biliary colic. His description of the disease includes colic, kidney stones, paralysis, encephalopathy, and cachexia (wasting). Although he suspected the wine of Poitou as one cause, there is no indication he considered contaminants in the wine to be responsible. Since Citois' description of the colic of Poitou represented the most authoritative view for a century and a half, his work is quoted extensively in a translation prepared by Michael Sollenberger.

> At almost the same time, or at least around 1572, when that new star in Cassiopeia was discovered, not without the secret understanding of God, to the extreme marvel of all astrologers, a new pain arose, Colic, called Bilious, because of the most bitter tortures from bile, as it was believed, and it lingers even yet. The one whose body it attacks, just as if struck by a star, it suddenly flings him down from his former condition, a pallor discolors his countenance, his limbs are numbed with cold, the strength grows faint, the spirit restless, the body disquieted, there is incessant wakefulness, swoonings, and rather frequent heartburn, appetite is ruined, there is continual nausea, belching, vomiting, and leek-green and often rusty-colored bile. And frequently gasping wears down the sick wretch, unquenchable thirst, distressing painful urination, and what very often occurs—a [kidney] stone. The area from ribs to groin is on

fire, without fever. Yet the chief symptom of the whole evil is the sharpest and most excruciating pain of the belly, intestines, loins, groin, and private parts.

After so many hardships, marvelous to say, the sick person, now believing that he is getting better, as he certainly does whenever the stomach pains have abated, begins to perceive distinctly that his arms and feet are being weakened. Movement of the elbows, hands, legs, and feet is lost. Some epileptic convulsions precede this paralysis in most cases, and once they destroyed many, but now, fewer and fewer.

After several months, their strength having come back to their limbs, they are again seen in the villages, just like ghosts, or statues, sallow, dirty, thin, with curved hands that hang down from their own weight, and only with effort are raised to the mouth and to the upper parts, and with feet that do not seem to be their own, and the muscles of the legs having been adapted for a ridiculous, if not pitiable gait. . . .

Yet, sometimes we vex the stomach with a concoction of difficult and undigestible foods. And no less noxious are pungent and bitter things, which sort of things are all raw fruit, and unripe fruit. All astringent foods, heavy, earthy, and flatulence-producing, which since the belly cannot digest and consume them, it changes on its own into flatulence and corrupt humors of various sorts. Of this sort indeed are our Pictonian wines, especially the recent ones (pp. 169–71).

Citois considered the colic of Poitou a kind of acid indigestion. Despite his failure to identify lead as the cause, his description of colica Pictonum gained well-deserved attention as a symptom complex. The torture of the colic was engraved on the popular mind. "One suffers such violent inward Contractions," wrote John Purcell in 1714, "that it feels to him, as if his Guts and Bowels were surrounded and pull'd together with Cords" (612, p. 2). This graphic image was used by George Cruikshank in 1819 (fig. 3); a picture on the wall depicts the cause of colic as drinking. Purcell was aware that "the Cholick frequently ends in a Palsey, or Epilepsy, sometimes in Gout" (p. 3), but was less sanguine about etiology. He listed 19 causes including "Crudities and Indigestions, sharp, sower, corrosive &c. and under this Head are to be compris'd as Causes of the Cholick, all sower and sharp Wines, Syders, Beer, Liquors, Fruits, &c." (p. 34), but also "Toads, Serpents, Lizards &c" (p. 44).

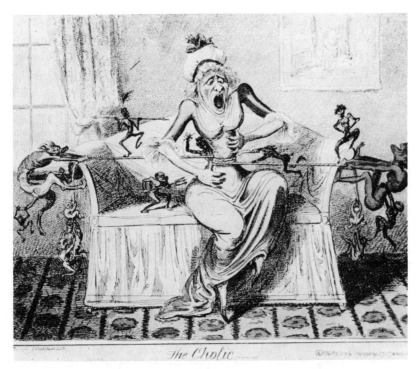

*3. The Cholic, engraved by George Cruikshank, 1819. From the collection of
the National Library of Medicine.*

In 1656, Samuel Stockhausen noted that colic was a regular occurrence among workers in the lead mines in Goslar (714). This remarkable physician recognized that the complaints of the villagers of Poitou were identical to the metallic colic of miners, an affliction the miners termed "Hüttenkatze." According to H. J. Siemens, this name was used "because the intolerable excruciations sometimes compels the one ailing to imitate the circumgyrations of a rabid cat" (685, p. 26). Stockhausen noted further that saturnine colic was sometimes followed by gout. He had the genius to challenge humoral theory by proposing a verifiable cause of the disease. Rejecting the fifteenth-century explanations of Ellenbog, Stockhausen embarked on deductive reasoning pervaded with intuitive epidemiology. He did not, however, attempt experimental proof of his theory.

In 1671, Johann Jacob Wepfer condemned the use of litharge and sugar of lead to "correct" the wines of Alsace and Wurttemberg (799). Writing of "paresis after colic from wine," Wepfer attributed colic, convulsions, paralysis, gout, suppression of the urine, and nephritis to that malignant practice. To detect tainted wine, Wepfer added six to twelve drops of "rectified oil of vitriol" (sulfuric acid) to three or four ounces of wine. The appearance of a milklike curd signified the presence of lead. While the delayed consequences of the adulterant (gout and nephritis) were forgotten for over a century, the acute symptoms of contaminated wine became the focus of a local furor. In 1691 John Jacob Francis Vicarius acknowledged Wepfer's important discovery and verified the dire consequences to the community (765).

In 1696 Eberhard Gockel, a distinguished physician of Ulm, suffered from colic after sharing wine with the monks of Wengen. Gockel subsequently published the monastic recipes to "correct" wine with litharge that had caused his grief (223). Acknowledging his debt to Stockhausen, he proceeded to survey the wines of the Neckar valley. Using a few drops of sulfuric acid, he again verified Stockhausen's theory. The addition of litharge to wine was clearly incriminated as the cause of the colica Pictonum prevalent in Ulm from 1694 to 1696. Gockel's assay for lead has been shown to be sufficiently sensitive to detect about 10 mg of lead per liter. Given the recipes detailed by Gockel, Eisinger estimates that the seventeenth century wines of Wurttemberg contained 16 mg of lead per liter while those encountered by Columella in ancient Rome contained almost twice as much (222, 223).

A gruesome demonstration of the fatal effects of lead was described by Johann Jacob Brunner in 1688 (102). Brunner claimed to have given an unfortunate victim, "one scrupple of white powder of litharge." After eleven hours of ghastly abdominal pains, convulsions, and bloody vomit, the subject expired. A postmortem examination revealed only redness of the intestines. Brunner reported neither the circumstances of this experiment, nor how the victim was selected. It is, in fact, doubtful that this catastrophic investigation actually took place, since such a minute dose of lead oxide (135 mg) would not be expected to produce so calamitous a result. The danger of leaded wine was, nevertheless, well recognized in Germany.

In Ulm, heads were severed for adulterating wines. By the end of the century, reports of the consequences of lead-contaminated wine were circulating more widely (518), but protective measures were, at best, irregular. Medical communications were sparse, theory confounded fact, and anecdotes displaced observation. Warnings faded with distance and went largely unnoticed outside of Germany. Deliberate suppression of the scandalous truth by those whose livelihoods were threatened seems likely (223). Even Samuel Stockhausen's nephew, Philip, presenting his medical dissertation to his learned uncle, failed to note that the colic of Poitou had the same cause as the metallic colic of miners (713).

Physicians and patients alike were more interested in cures than causes, but consistency in treatment was as remote as consistency in diagnosis. Glowing testimonials abounded for every conceivable remedy. Amulets had the sanction of long tradition. Robert Burton recalled that "a Wolfs dung born with one helps the Cholick" (106, p. 245), but could not condone advice "to swallow a bullet of lead" (p. 249) to relieve constipation.

During his travels in the Orient, Theopholus Bonet learned that burning of flesh was an excellent remedy (78).

> In the violent pain of the Colick (such as rages horribly all Asia over, and often kills the Patient with unspeakable Torments, or frequently leaveth a Palsie in the hand and feet behind it) the Portuguese use this Remedy; they stand barefoot on a hot Iron (instead whereof I should use Artemisial Down, with less pain, and perhaps more benefit) till the burnt part hiss, and they feel pain, upon which they presently find ease, otherwise they are counted incurable (p. 37).

An early advocate of flammable cures, Sir William Temple could nevertheless recommend more conservative remedies. "Garlick is of great Virtue in all Cholicks," he proclaimed in "An Essay Upon Health and Long Life," ". . . a great Strengthener of the Stomach upon Decays of Appetite and Indigestion: And I believe, is (if at least there be any Such) a Specific Remedy of the Gout" (738, p. 179).

The preeminent Hermann Boerhaave recommended bleeding, clysters, opiates and, if all else failed, treatment "by fomentations of the like kind applied all over the Belly, and chiefly the Application of young live, hot and found Animals; such as Puppies or Kittens" (77, p. 149). The efficacy of puppies derived, according to folklore, from their empathy for human suffering; the pain was absorbed by the willing canine host (223). Robert James on the other hand, preferred chicken soup (396). "As for that terrible convulsive-spasmodical Colic, called Saturnine . . . which afflicts workmen employed in Smelting or otherwise manufacturing of Lead and torments them to a most violent Degree, there is no better preservative, invented, than taking some fat Broth in the morning" (p. 247).

In his *Bath Memoires*, Robert Pierce recalled many years of successful medical practice at Britain's favorite spa in the seventeenth century

(603). According to Pierce, the waters of Bath were equally effective taken externally or internally in the treatment of palsies. To an extensive roster of patients he had cured of this malady, Pierce adds the names of travelers from the American Plantations in Barbados. "All, and many more, for the same Loss of Limbs, after the Belly-ach (for so long they term this Pictonic Cholick in those parts) were here relieved," he reported, "if not perfectly restored to Strength" (p. 101).

Half a century later, William Oliver concurred with Pierce in recommending Bath waters for colica Pictonum then so prevalent in the West Indies (565). The mineral waters remained a popular remedy for lead poisoning even as the true cause became known. George Baker quotes his colleague, Dr. Andrew of Exeter, on the virtues of Bath waters "being esteemed by us the most effectual remedy, both internally and externally used" (31, p. 201). From 1751 to 1746, 1,053 patients were admitted to the Bath Hospital with palsy; 237 with "Palsies from Cyder and Bilious Cholica." The Bath Waters reportedly cured 80 percent irrespective of etiology (133).

The value of Bath waters in the treatment of lead poisoning is doubtful since the pipes and cisterns from which the waters flowed were fashioned from lead (250, 435, 565). In Roman times, the baths were lined with massive sheets of lead (554). The visible corrosion of the plumbing made it probable that these highly praised waters were more likely to induce than alleviate saturnism. The methods available to Baker were not sufficiently sensitive to detect the minute traces of lead dissolved in the water, but refinements in technique soon made it apparent that much of Britain's water supply was, indeed, contaminated (435). To supplement such unassuming therapies, inventive physicians sought more dramatic treatment for Dr. Baker's celebrated colic. Christopher Pemberton devised a specific splint for lead palsy which he made available to the public in 1806 (fig. 4, [596]).

In seventeenth-century England cider production evolved into a prodigious industry. By 1765, hard cider consumption ranged between 2.5 and 5 pints per year for every man, woman, and child. Consumption did not reach comparable levels again until the 1970s (704). In Devonshire the taste for cider was exceeded only by the appetite for selling it. When Parliament voted a tax on the local brew the citizens of Devon mustered a committee to demand repeal (154).

Despite its enormous popularity, cider's reputation was tarnished. In 1703 John Philips' poem "Cyder" contained the lines (486):

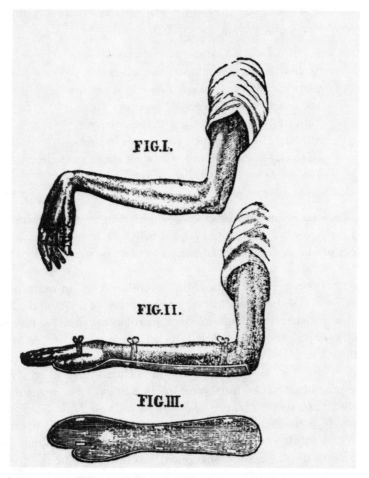

4. Forearm splint devised by C. R. Pemberton in 1806 for the treatment of lead palsy (596).

The Must, of palid hue, declares the soil
Devoid of spirit; wretched he, that quaffs
Such wheyish liquors; oft with colic pangs,
With pungent colic pangs distress he'll roar,
And toss, and turn, and curse th'unwholsome draught.

(p. 35)

Cider, in this grim song, is the cause of "joint racking gout" and "pining atrophy," as well as the colic. Abstinence is the only hope (602). Invoking

Vulcan, the Roman god of fire and metalworking, Philips deplores the adulteration of cider.

> But, this I warn thee and shall always warn,
> No heterogeneous mixtures use, as some
> With watery turnips have debased their wines
> Too frugal, nor let the crude humours dance
> In heated brass, steaming with fire intense;
> Although Devonia much commends the use
> Of strengthening Vulcan; with their native strength
> Thy wines sufficient, other aid refuse.

(p. 65)

It was widely known that cider could be dangerous to health (659, 683). Yet, over a century later, a good bellyache from cider was still a subject of humor (fig. 5) in England, and of alarm in the United States (107).

In 1703, Musgrave described the Devonshire colic in more prosaic terms. He noted that this affliction was the result of drinking hard cider and was associated with a number of neurologic symptoms. Unfamiliar with the works of Stockhausen and Gockel, Musgrave, too, failed to identify the cause of the colic, but he did observe that gout was its frequent companion (353). Two decades later John Huxham recorded a recurrence of epidemic colic in Devonshire. In *A small Treatise on the Devonshire Colic which was very epidemic in the year 1724*, Huxham unknowingly delineated the neurologic manifestations arising from lead and noted that arthritis often accompanied the more acute symptoms (390). "Commonly the Rheumatism succeeded the Colic, the Colic the Rheumatism and thus alternately tormented the miserable Patients, the Disease now being translated to the Limbs, now to the bowels" (p. 9).

The rheumatism Huxham associated with the colic was gout. "Nor are there any where so many, even amongst the very common People, as in the County of Devon, most famous for Cyder, that are afflicted with the Gout" (p. 17). Cider was not, however, all bad. Though it caused the colic and the gout, Huxham was convinced cider would cure the scurvy (which was true) and leprosy (which was not).

In the absence of obvious lead absorption the cause of the symptoms remained obscure. Huxham ascribed the Devonshire colic to the weather and to the "tartar" of cider but primarily to the plethora of apples. According to Huxham, even the hogs were made sick by overfeeding with

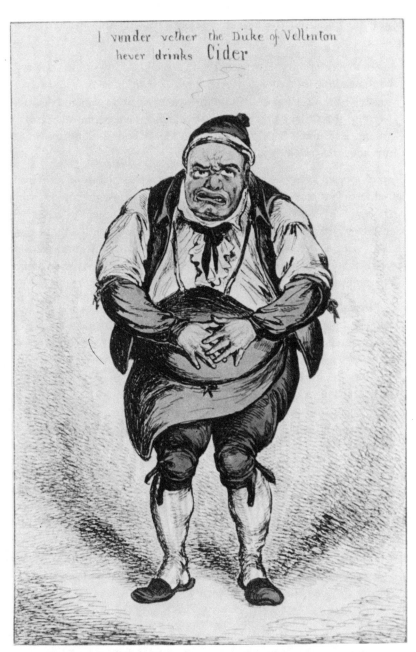

5. *Abdominal pain was the* Blessing of Cheap Cider *as engraved by William Heath in 1850. These "gripes" were not necessarily dry. From the author's collection.*

apples. He chastised the farmers for impiety, who thus wasted "kind Providence."

> Some more pious perhaps, but not very sober, daily swilled down whole Gallons of Cyder, nay even hired People to drink it, lest forsooth God's Blessings should be thrown away; and again and again filled up the Casks as they drank it out. A sacrifice perhaps acceptable to a drunken Bacchus, but by no Means approved by the Supreme Father of Gods and Men! (p. 13).

Despite careful observation, Huxham could not separate casual from causal associations. George Baker scoffed at his inconsistencies (31).

The reason cider caused the colic remained the subject of extensive speculation and little insight. But the foundations for identifying the connection with lead were slowly being constructed. In 1736 the works of Stephen Francis Geoffroy were published posthumously. This outstanding French pharmacist, chemist, and physician observed of lead (297):

> From the excellent Virtues of this Metal, Paracelsus called it the "Fourth Pillar of Physic." In itself, or without Preparation, it is cooling, incrassating, repellent, absorbent, and lenient. It is believed to be an Enemy of Venery, and undoubtedly calms Effervescences in the Blood, and checks the Progress of Inflammations, but is very destructive to the Nerves. Taken inwardly, it loads the Stomach, gripes, and stops the Excretion of both Feces and Urine. It brings on Spasms and Tremblings, Difficulty of Breathing, and Suffocations; which direful Effects many have felt by drinking Wine recovered by Litharge after it has grown sowre (p. 243).

By the middle of the eighteenth century the consequences of plumbism were well, if not widely, known. But identifying lead poisoning arising from the contamination of food and drink was still difficult. Despite the similarity of symptoms, the cause of the colic and palsy arising from adulterated beverages was not generally recognized as identical to that which produced these symptoms in lead workers. Thus John Wesley's *Primitive Physic* contains the following entries (801):

> 44. A Nervous Colic*.
> 204. Use the Cold Bath daily for a Month:
> 205. Or, take Quicksilver and Aqua Sulphurata daily for a month:
>   * This is frequently term'd the dry Belly-Ach. It often
>   continues several Days, with Urine, and obstinate Costivness.

45. Colic from the Fumes of Lead, or White-Lead, Verdigrease, &c.

206. In the Fit drink melted Butter, and then vomit with warm water:

208. To prevent or cure. Breakfast daily on fat Broth, and use Oil of sweet Almonds frequently and largely.

209. Smelters of Metals, Plumbers, &c may be in a good Measure preserved from the poisonous Fumes that surround them, by breathing thro' Cloth or Flannel Mufflers twice or thrice doubled, dipt in a Solution of Sea Salt, or Salt of Tartar and then dried. These Mufflers might also be of Use in many similar Cases

(pp. 52–53).

Concurring with Boerhaave, the founder of Methodism recognized a third condition of unknown etiology with similar symptoms: "The Gout of the Stomach." For what he supposed to be still another separate entity, "Palsy from working with white Lead or Verdigrease," Wesley prescribed "warm Baths and a Milk Diet" (p. 109).

Traditionally, noxious air had been held responsible for the colic (12, 146, 390). Until the middle of the nineteenth century, meticulous records were kept in order to identify correlations between the direction of winds, the degree of humidity, and the prevalence of disease. For the ubiquitous febrile diseases such etiologic considerations were forgotten after the discovery of infectious agents at the end of the nineteenth century. While meteorologic considerations seem ludicrous to the modern reader, there was in fact some rational basis upon which such correlations might be made with lead colic. There is reason to believe that the manifestations of lead poisoning are to some extent determined by the weather.

The tendency of Devonshire colic to occur in autumn was explained by George Baker in terms of the apple harvest. Since apples ripen in late summer, by fall they tend to be both overabundant and overripe. Lead acetate would have been particularly useful in preventing spoilage of cider in the heat of early autumn.

In children, too, lead poisoning occurs more frequently in summer than any other season (22, 557). It had long been suspected that the prevalence of lead poisoning in tropical climates might be related to the interaction of sunlight, vitamin D, and calcium with lead metabolism. Milk and calcium have repeatedly been reported to protect from lead poisoning, but the interaction between lead and vitamin D is clearly quite complex (655). Since vitamin D activity is stimulated by ultraviolet light, there may be some biological justification for the ancient astrologic view; climatic conditions may influence the expression of saturnism. While correlation is not causation, a cause for correlation can sometimes be found.

Chemical techniques to support such observations were soon devised. The methods for detection of lead in liquids used by Wepfer and Gockel in the seventeenth century had won few imitators but in the eighteenth century, the German apothecary and follower of Stahl, Caspar Neuman, rediscovered the phenomenon. Neuman reacted arsenous sulfide (then known as orpiment or auripigment) with lead to form a dark precipitate. "And hence we are furnished with means for discovering the dangerous fraud of impregnating wines with Litharge. If the Wine, on being mixed with the solution of Auripigment, acquires a brownish red or blackish colour, we may be sure it has suffered that abuse" (550, p. 155).

Neuman's method for detecting lead was published in 1740, several years after his death, and was translated into English in 1759. His teachings were well known to aspiring chemists, but more romantic uses of auripigment attracted greater attention. The yellow stone, when powdered, made a pleasing gold paint for artists and invisible ink for intriguers (374).

The black precipitate formed by hydrogen sulfide and lead promoted creative exploitation well into the nineteenth century. M. L. Byrn found that bathing in a solution of hydrogen sulfide had salutary effects in cases of lead colic, which effects were evident by the blackening of the patients' skin (108). Others used lead sulfide to restore the luster of youth to graying locks, at the same time risking their lives. Hall's Vegetable Sicilian Hair Renewer, for example, contained 15 mg of lead per gram (560). Today's Grecian Formula 9 (372) and Youthair Creme bring the same glories of youth to modern graybeards. The practical applications of chemistry to medicine encounter more resistance than do the frivolous.

It was George Baker who impressed the significance of insidious lead poisoning on modern medical consciousness. Unlike Gockel's efforts in 1697, Baker's observation received immediate international attention. The thoroughness of his inquiries, the elegance of his logic, but mainly his compelling application of chemistry to medicine made Baker's writings a landmark in the history of medicine. Like a detective in a maze of diversions, Baker systematically unraveled the cause of the Devonshire colic. He cited earlier authorities when appropriate, absorbed criticisms when sound, but was never diverted by vested interests or conventional wisdom that contradicted his observations. His work was a model of epidemiology and science touched with eloquence.

When Baker read "An Essay concerning the Cause of the Endemial Colic of Devonshire" to the College of Physicians in 1767, he began with a memorable admonition to scholars (30).

> A very small acquaintance with the writings of physicians is sufficient to convince us, that much labour and ingenuity has been most unprofitably bestowed on the investigation of remote and obscure causes; while those, which are immediate and obvious, and which must necessarily be admitted, as soon as discovered, have too frequently been overlooked and disregarded. . . . We have now learned, not to indulge in visioning speculations, but to attend closely to nature. We observe diseases in themselves, and trace the powers of medicines in their effects on the human body; and experiment is the great basis of our reasoning (pp. 175–76).

Baker then reviewed the work of Citois, Musgrave, and Huxham noting that each had described a similar syndrome but had failed to correctly identify the cause (31).

> But, lead itself being certainly of such a nature, as to be abundantly answerable for all the ill effects complained of from the cyder, my thoughts were naturally carried to the search of it; and well might I expect to find it, in some way or another combined with that liquor.
>
> No author, whom I have had an opportunity of consulting has given any information of having conceived the same suspicion with myself, except only the anonymous author of *Examen d'un livre qui a pour titre T. Tronchin de colica Pictonum.* This writer indeed hints in a cursory manner. . . . It is evident, however, from what he afterwards says, . . . that he was very far from having formed a settled opinion of this subject (p. 189).

The anonymous author cited by Baker had good reason to remain unknown; this French physician accused Tronchin of flagrant plagiarism, abysmal ignorance, and a miserable literary style. Tronchin was a favorite pupil of Boerhaave, personal physician to Voltaire, and one of the most successful practitioners in eighteenth-century Paris (284). Tronchin had listed lead among a kaleidoscope of causes of colica Pictonum (752). The abusive monograph by "un Médecin de Paris," ultimately attributed to P.

Bouvart (12, 30, 296), while demolishing the contributions of Tronchin, reveals Bouvart to have understood the cause of the colic of Poitou a decade before Baker. Bouvart wrote (83):

> M. Tronchin not only makes a marked differentiation between metal colic and vegetable colic but he imagines six other species of colic whose original causes according to him are badly cured fevers, gout, rheumatism, arrested perspiration, melancholy and passions of the soul.
>
> The colic of potters, painters, lead workers, enamelers, lapidaries and gilders of metals and many other artisans is the same disease. One can also add the disease of green wine or wines turning sour which by a fraud worthy of the most severe punishment, certain tavernkeepers sweeten with litharge. It is possible that the wines spoken of by Citois and the cider spoken of by M. Huxham may have been, without their having been able to discover it, altered with litharge or with some other similar substance. What is certain is that the colic in question has been epidemic in the countries where they drink Rhein and Moselle wines. These wines are often deficient by reason of immaturity and merchants have for a long time altered them with litharge (p. 7).

Although Bouvart's scurrilous attack was directed at Tronchin, his quarrel was actually with eighteenth-century French scholasticism. Like his contemporaries, Bouvart could not confidently exclude all of the reputed causes of the colic. This hesitancy was undoubtedly warranted, since much of what was diagnosed as the colic of Poitou was probably not due to lead. Dysentery was still included under this rubric. It was not until after Baker proved the etiology of the Devonshire colic that the various other intestinal syndromes could be differentiated. Vague classification perpetuated conceptual ambiguity. The precise definition of disease requires exact diagnostic methods. Under the circumstances, Bouvart's rebuttal of Tronchin showed remarkable acumen—an inspired guess. Baker surely underestimated Bouvart.

Tronchin's treatise on colica Pictonum triggered a lively debate in which polemic dominated insight. Led by de Haen (344), who suspected but could not prove the lead etiology, a multiplicity of causes prevailed. Apart from Bouvart, the thinking of the Parisian physicians was as fuzzy as it was dogmatic. The physicians were more concerned with theories of therapy than with pathogenesis. The source of the best mineral water was of greater interest than was the cause of the disease. In a series of papers appearing between 1762 and 1765, Bordeu, the leading proponent of the "vitalistic" theory of disease, analyzed available data on the colic of Poitou (79). According to this theory, living matter differs fundamentally from inanimate matter. The mystical concept of a vital spirit rendered simple chemical causes almost inconceivable. Despite his familiarity with painters' colic and his case reports of plumbers' colic and palsy, Bordeu could not extract a single etiology from the maze of information.

Among the Parisian theoreticians, Bouvart, alone, proposed lead as the sole cause of colica Pictonum. In footnotes to the second editions of their respective works, Bouvart and Baker each claimed priority for recognizing lead as the cause of the colic of Poitou. Expressing restrained enthusiasm for George Baker's contribution, Bouvart wrote (83):

> Here, then, are my suspicions borne out and fully justified by these observations. Mr. Baker has demonstrated in 1767 the fact which I had only conjectured in 1757; thus I owe him thanks for giving the proof of what I had imagined. But let him not dispute with my conjecture the right of ten year priority which it has over his! (p. 10).

To which Baker responded in a footnote to *his* second edition (35):

> I am desirous to pay all due honour to this learned and astute physician: but in the present case, I cannot acknowledge the justice of his pretensions. . . . Having again read over his pamphlet, I found no reason to alter my original sentiment: I must therefore demur to the claim of prior occupancy (p. 433).

Bouvart lost considerable ground in the debate by altering the text of his second edition, a doctoring effort which did not escape Baker's attention. Baker concluded his footnote by pointing out that such polemics are beneath his dignity. "From hence it manifestly appears, that, in the year 1758, this author had really conceived some doubts. . . . But let me not engage further in a controversy so entirely uninteresting, and so unimportant!" (p. 136).

Arguments about the cause of the colic of Poitou nevertheless continued unabated on both sides of the English Channel. In the course of the dispute, the etiology of the colic was narrowed to two categories: vegetable and mineral (metallic). Metal colic was considered to include mercury, antimony, arsenic, and copper, as well as lead. Too many contradictory observations had become ensconced in medical lore to be resolved into a single etiology. In attempting to explain all, they explained nothing. The characteristic features of lead colic were lost in a profusion of anecdotal reports. The quarrel was endless and hopeless. Only Baker reached beyond caustic comment to resolve conjecture with experiment.

The arid debate in France served to confound the issues even after George Baker had provided the solution. Samuel Tissot, fellow of the Royal Society of London and of the Physico-Medical Academy of Basel, was unpersuaded by Baker's unitary explanation (748). "I shall not presume to resolve the controversy," he averred in 1773, "but should myself be of the opinion, that some wines, poisonous substances, and the scurvy, are the three causes which excite cholics, followed by a paralytic disorder: and that no other causes are to be allowed" (pp. 200–201). The insular French academicians were less than eager to give Baker his due.

The absurdity of these quarrels reached ever new heights with claims of therapeutic priority. Bordeu contended that treatment of metal colic had been perfected at L'Hôpital de la Charité in 1602. The composition of this secret remedy imported from Italy was transmitted by word of mouth among the hospital's monks. By the beginning of the eighteenth century it was primarily a mixture of antimony and sugar (730). Apparently late revisions of this famed formula did not diminish its potency.

Almost a century later lead colic from cider was still familiar in France (134, 566). In an 1833 lithograph very reminiscent of Cruikshank's earlier print (fig. 3), Daumier satirized the agony of the colic in a Frenchman of considerably more elegance than his English predecessor (fig. 6). To a Frenchman the ultimate humiliation occurred when the colic interfered with his connubial obligations (fig. 7). In French parodies, the physician attempting to treat colic was almost as ludicrous as when treating the gout (fig. 8).

While George Baker was not alone in suspecting that lead was the cause of colica Pictonum, his contribution was decisive. Departing from dogma, he moved medicine closer to the scientific method; experiment became "the great basis of our reasoning." The educated guess went out of style, or at least went into competition with verifiable fact. Rather than insisting that observation fit time-honored theory, physicians began to adapt theory to observation.

Baker was well aware of the many sources of lead in cider including: cisterns, glazed earthenware, cider-press covers, rollers, repair patches, troughs, and linings of various parts of the cider presses. In a subsequent communication to the College of Physicians, he reviewed other sources of lead poisoning including cosmetics, shot, paint, glazed vessels, pewter, and water pipes (34). Of deliberate adulteration Baker wrote:

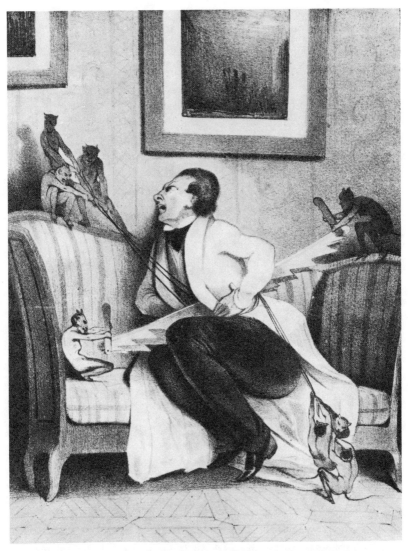

6. La Colique *was as excruciating to this elegant Frenchman as to Cruikshank's more mundane Englishwoman (fig. 3). Lithograph by C. Ramelet after H. Daumier, 1833.*

I had indeed been informed, that it is the practice of some farmers, in managing this weak cyder, made early in the year, before the apples are ripe, to put a leaden weight into the cask, in order to prevent the liquor from being sour; and that this cyder is the common drink of their servants and laborers. But I was willing to be-

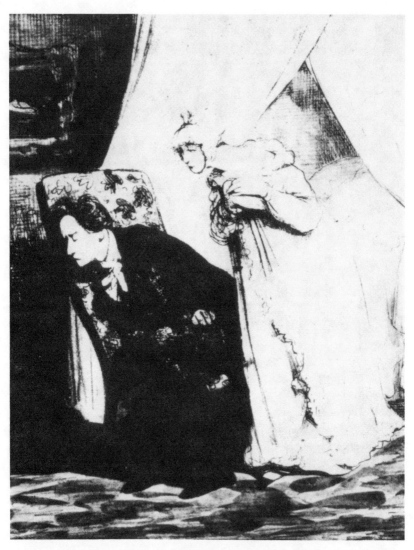

7. Avoir la colique le jour de ses noces *[Colic on his wedding night]. The ultimate humiliation as depicted in a lithograph from the series* Les Petits Malheurs du bonheur *by P. Gavarni in 1838.*

lieve, that such a pernicious method of adulteration (a crime, which in both France and Germany is punished by death) was not often practiced by our countrymen. That it is not practiced with any consciousness of the mischief of it, I still hope and believe. But it is certainly common, with dealers in cyder, when the liquor frets

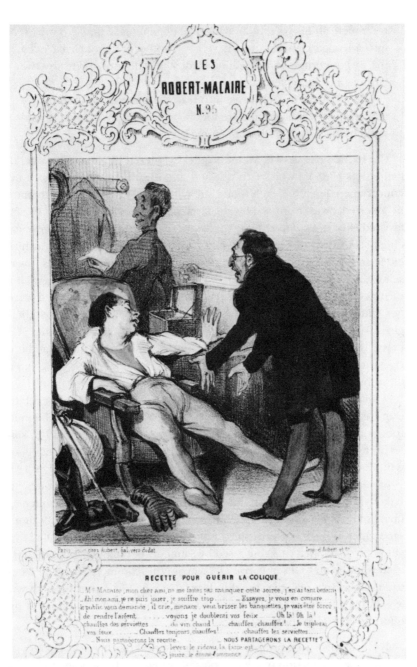

8. Recette pour guérir la colique *[Recipe to cure the colic]. Drawn in the style of Daumier, from the series* Robert-Macaire, *this sufferer from the colic has reason to regret his latest debauch. Published by Aubert, 1839.*
From the author's collection.

too much, and is thereby in danger of becoming acetous, to rack it into a leaden cistern. And I have good authority to add, that even the use of cerusse in correcting acidity, is well known both by the farmers and merchants. . . .

Indeed, there is great reason to fear, that pernicious methods of adulterating vinous liquors are too well known, and too much practiced in every part of this kingdom (pp. 208–15).

The battle lines drawn, seconds quickly entered the field for a duel of pamphlets (788). In order to promote the health and prosperity of his countrymen, Francis Geach took issue with Baker's claims. "No litharge," he asserted, "was ever used by any farmer in Devon" (295, p. 13). Geach favored Huxham's acid-residue theory. He cited the inability of two local chemists (More and Cookworthy by name) to detect lead in Devonshire cider and defended the multiplicity of causes with logic as thin as it was self-righteous. Lead, he claimed, could not be the "universal cause" because colic was not the "universal effect." Many who were afflicted were not cider drinkers at all. "Chlorotic" females, who maintained their girlish figures by drinking vinegar, also suffered from pallor, colic, and palsy. Acids regularly induced convulsions in children, he noted, and unripe fruit brought on the gout. Lead, Geach concluded, must be given a clean bill of health.

William Saunders issued a prompt retort on Baker's behalf. After rebutting Geach's spurious arguments, he observed, "There appears to be in it, too evident marks of ignorance, for us, to suspect mere wilfull misinterpretation; and at the same time there appears too evident marks of wilfull misinterpretation, for us, to suspect only ignorance" (669, p. 18).

In his rejoinder, Geach renewed his attack on the weak points in Baker's work: the specificity and sensitivity of the lead assay were open to question as was Baker's sampling technique. There were about six thousand cider presses in Devonshire and rigorous random sampling had not yet been developed (12). Accused by Saunders of building "hypothetical castles in the air," Geach parried, "To avoid this common fault, you Doctor, more wisely chose to build in lead" (296, p. 26). Admiring such wit less in his adversary than in himself, Geach completed his argument by offering "a little friendly advice."

Never expect to advance either your medical or chemical character, by an affectation of wit and pleasantry. Levity ill becomes a physician, who ought to be a sober enquirer after truth. Mirth, which may set a few jovial club companions in a roar, will be hardly under-

stood, and not at all relished by the plain and honest farmers of Devon; who (if this doctrine be credited) must never expect to pay
their rents from the produce of their orchards (p. 52).

Thomas Alcock, a "Reverend Ecclesiastic," joined the defense of Devonshire cider, to "put an End to this Leaden Controversey" (12, p. 5).
Admitting that he occasionally profited from the sale of cider, Alcock proposed an alternate cause of the colic: "an irregular Gout, may rather produce, or contribute to produce, and increase, this Distemper in such Sea-
sons, than this supposed solution of Lead" (p. 18). Alcock, too, was
unable to detect lead in cider. Any adulterant found by others, he assured
his readers, was introduced by the London distributors or by the inexplicable and unique addition of buckshot to Dr. Baker's samples. Acknowledging that Baker might appropriately have warned the public of
such dangers, the Reverend Alcock admonished Baker for impugning the
reputation of the blameless Devonshire farmers.

> But now by the Doctrines published in the *Essay, a very great
> and needless Expence may be incurred, by breaking up old
> Pounds and erecting new ones. . . .* Devonshire Cyder, notwith-
> standing the late great scarcity, is become a mere Drug at the Lon-
> don Market, and almost all Orders for that Liquor, are sent to Here-
> ford, as I foresaw and predicted (p. 82).

In another attempt to improve the position of Devonshire cider in the
slumping London market, one "Danmoniensis," declared that Baker had
perpetrated a gross injustice on local farmers. In those rare instances
where lead could be found in the cider of Devin it was mere accident,
"from the common Custom of shooting Thrushes, etc. off the Apple
Heaps in the Winter. All the Shots which do not lodge in the Birds are
stuck into the Apples" (179, p. 12). Lead shot lodged in apples seems an
unlikely source of poisoned cider, but a genuine threat existed in the cooking of game birds. In 1983 the menu of the Crusting Pipe Restaurant in
Covent Garden still alerted patrons to the "lead shot hazard" in its sump-
tuous "Game Pie." Baker was from time to time derided or ignored, but in
the end his analysis prevailed. Despite the local furor, the methods of cider
manufacturing were gradually modified to reduce lead contamination.

Following Baker's reports, the toxicology of lead took on new interest.
In *A Candid Examination of what has been Advanced as the Colic of
Poitou and Devonshire, with Remarks on the Most Probable and Experi-
ments Intended to Ascertain the True Causes of Gout,* James Hardy

reconciled the differences in Musgrave's and Baker's observations (353). He was the first to authoritatively confirm the view that gout was a consequence of lead poisoning. Hardy speculated that Hippocrates was probably familiar with lead colic because of the Greek practice of preparing wines in leaden vessels and of deliberately adding sugar of lead to stabilize and sweeten them. His own experiments showed that alcoholic beverages leached dangerous quantities of lead from glazed vessels. Hardy used a rather crude chemical technique for measuring lead in aqueous solutions which has recently been shown to be reliable only for lead concentrations over 1 mg/liter (774). Eighteenth-century methods for detecting lead in liquids were, nevertheless, ten times more sensitive than those of the previous century (223). Hardy suspected that the contamination of West India rum, like the Devonshire cider, arose from the glazes used on British export wares (353) which contained "one ounce of lead-ore to every quart in measure" (p. 43).

At least for a time, the lesson of the Devonshire colic was learned even by the ubiquitous "mountebanks and quacks" who practiced medicine in London. In an extensive treatise on the scurvy, gout, and diet distributed by Francis Spilsbury in order to sell his secret antimony-mercury cure, we find dire warnings of the gout resulting from "cyder standing in leaden vats, or in earthen pitchers glazes with lead" (702, p. 70). Unwilling to sacrifice his creative imagination to George Baker, Spilsbury preferred his own explanation for the colic arising from rum. Discoursing on "A Liquor Called Punch," he attributed the colic and gout, not to lead or acids, but to the sugar (703).

Skeptics abounded three decades after Baker's essays, and colic followed by palsy continued to plague the good farmers of Devon. Describing the traditional base of the rural economy, one agricultural expert attributed the colic to the effects of "rough and corrosive cider," noting that wool and cow dung had largely replaced lead for caulking the vats and presses (514). Economic need undermined Baker's observations.

In the absence of rigorous diagnostic criteria, it was difficult for physicians to keep track of the differences between "dry" and "wet" gripes. The presence of diarrhea seemed relatively inconsequential compared to the overwhelming abdominal pains. This clinical ambiguity is evident in a caricature of *The Dry Gripes or the Comforts of a Hot Summer* (fig. 9). While a woman (on the left) tipples a potentially lead-tainted beverage, the children (on the right), having consumed most of the cherries on the table, experience explosive diarrhea. Popular imagery conspired to make the clinician's task an arduous one.

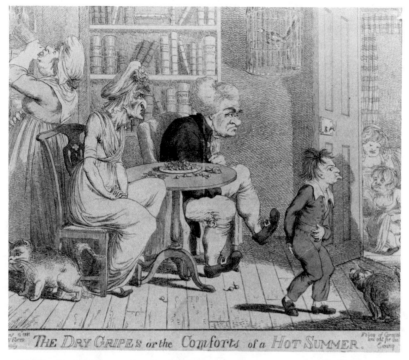

9. The Dry Gripes or the Comforts of a Hot Summer, *by G. M. Woodward,
1781. Spoiled cherries were more likely to produce wet gripes* (right) *than was
tippling* (left). *From the Clements C. Fry Collection, Yale Medical Library.*

The West India dry gripes provided Baker with evidence that acid
juices were not the cause of the colic. How could fruit juice cause the
disease, he asked (31),

> when it appears that Dr. Hillary greatly depended on it, for the cure
> of the dry-belly ach, in the West Indies? And lastly can we possibly
> allow, that a cause, similar in its nature to the acid of lemons, is pro-
> ductive of this disease in our country; after having been informed
> from the West Indies and the colonies of North America, that the
> juice of lemons and limes is not only much trusted for its cure, but
> that it is even esteemed to be a preservative from it? (p. 194).

In a later communication Baker expanded on the contribution of the
American colonies to his own understanding of the disease (32).

> My suspicions, concerning this subject, have been greatly con-
> firmed by the authority of Dr. Franklyn of Philadelphia. That gentle-

man informs me, that, at Boston about forty years ago, leaden worms were used for the distillation of rum. In consequence thereof, such violent disorders were complained of by the drinkers of new rum, that the government found it expedient to enact a law, forbidding the use of any worms, except such only as were made of pure block-tin. . . . They have used a pewter, containing a large proportion of lead.

Dr. Franklyn likewise informed me, that the colic of Poitou is not so frequent a disease in any of the colonies, as it was formerly; and that the reason, commonly assigned, is, that the people now drink their punch very weak in comparison with what they were formerly accustomed to; which used to be rum and water in equal quantities. He added, that they now also drink their punch, with more juice of fresh limes in it; and, as that juice, joined to certain laxative medicines, is at present their common remedy, when any are seized with the disease, so it is generally considered the best preservative against it (p. 286).

While not exactly rejecting anecdotal data, Baker was discriminating in choosing the source of such tales. He thus learned that the coiled metal tubing or "worm" used in the distilling apparatus was the source of lead in early New England rum.

In a letter to Benjamin Vaughn in 1786, Benjamin Franklin recalled his introduction to lead poisoning (270).

The first thing I remember of this kind was a general discourse in Boston, when I was a boy, of a complaint from North Carolina against New England rum, that it poisoned their people, giving them the dry bellyache with a loss of use of their limbs. The distilleries being examined on the occasion, it was found that several of them used leaden still heads and worms, and physicians were of the opinion, that the mischief was occasioned by the use of lead. The legislature of Massachusetts thereupon passed an act, prohibiting under several penalties, the use of such still heads and worms thereafter (p. 565).

In 1723 the Massachusetts Bay Colony had passed a law entitled, "An Act for Preventing Abuses in Distilling of Rum and Other Strong Liquors with Lead Heads of Pipes." Section I of the act stated (251):

That no person whatsoever shall make use of any such leaden heads or worms, for the future; and that whosoever shall presume to distil, or draw off any spirits or strong liquors thro' such leaden heads or worms, upon legal conviction thereof before any of his majest[y][ie]'s courts of record, shall forfeit and pay a fine of one hundred pounds (p. 577).

Unfortunately, no record of the legislative debate which preceded enactment of the law has been found (261). Whether enforcement of the Lead-Rum Act was effective in detoxifying "good old New England rum," is similarly unrecorded. Vast quantities of molasses continued to be distilled in New England throughout the eighteenth century. This enterprise was the economic backbone of the colonies and the currency of the slave trade. Legal constraints on rum manufacture did not impede the burgeoning triangular trade in molasses, rum, and slaves which tied New England to the West Indies and to Africa. The only impediment to the growing colonial prosperity was the payment of taxes to England. According to Charles William Taussig, the Molasses Act of 1733 gave more impetus to the American Revolution than either the tea trade or the Stamp Tax (732). Nor did the legal restrictions on lead worms restrain the infusion of rum punch into the life of the emerging nation. "The social and political aspect of rum and the Rebellion was to be found in the licensed houses and taverns," Taussig has noted, "for it was in those places of conviviality, carousing and caressing, that our republic was conceived" (p. 70).

Franklin was aware of lead colic at least as early as his sixteenth year. While serving as temporary editor of his brother's *New England Courant* in 1722, the following announcement appeared in that newspaper (488):

> For the Good of the Public, a certain Person hath a secret Medicine which cures the Gravil and Cholick immediately, and Dry Belly Ach in little Time; and restores the Use of the limbs again, (tho of never so long continuance) and is excellent for the Gout. Enquire of Mr. Samuel Gerrish, Bookseller, near the Brick Meeting House over against the Town House in Boston. N.B. The Poor who are not able to pay for it may have it gratis (p. 575).

The dry bellyache was by no means new to the American colonies. "Of the Colic of the People of Poictiers," Sydenham had recorded, "this is a kind of colic which ordinarily degenerates into a palsy, and a total loss of the motion of the hands and feet. Riverius described it under this name. It is a common disorder in the Caribbee islands, where it seizes abundance of persons" (723, p. 442). In 1684 the colonist John Clayton wrote to the illustrious Robert Boyle, a sufferer from gout, and founder of modern chemistry (138):

> The Distemper of the Colick that is predominant and has miserable sad effects. It begins with violent gripes wch. declining takes away the use of the limbs. Their fingers stand stiffly bent, the hands of some hang as if they were loose at the wrists from the arms, they are sceletons so meagre and leane that a consumption might seeme a fatning to them, cruelly are they distracted with a flatus, and at length those that seemingly recover are oft troubled with a sort of gout (p. 213).

There were few physicians in the American colonies in the eighteenth century; the business of health care fell largely to educated laymen. Provincial practice was nevertheless surprisingly current, fed by a continuous infusion from continental sources. The celebrated minister Cotton Mather was as erudite on the secrets of medicine as of God. Between sermons he prepared a truly learned manuscript on medicine which was delayed some two and a half centuries in publication. Writing on the "Dry-Belly-Ache" in 1723, Mather recommended snakeweed noting, "The physicians in the West Indies use it as a specific for the Dry-Belly-ache" (516, p. 220).

In 1745 Benjamin Franklin published a pamphlet by Thomas Cadwalader, then residing in Trenton, New Jersey, entitled *An Essay on the West-India Dry-Gripes with the Method of Preventing and Curing that Cruel Distemper to which is Added an Extraordinary Case in Physick* (111). Cadwalader was a close associate of Franklin in Philadelphia. He was among the first four consultants appointed to the Pennsylvania Hospital. A scholar credited with teaching the first course in medicine in the Western Hemisphere, Cadwalader had ample opportunity to see the "dry-gripes" in Philadelphia where Jamaican rum was extremely popular, and tableware was commonly made of pewter with high lead content (253, 488). Cadwalader recognized the similarity of the West India dry gripes to colica Pictonum. However, he did more than simply recount the classic descriptions of the colic of Poitou. Cadwalader saw that Citois' explanation of etiology could not be correct. In rejecting Citois' theory that the colic was caused by acidic fruit juices, he lay the groundwork for Baker's later inquiries.

> Thus Negroes in some Parts of the West-Indies, ease the excessive Pains in the Dry-Gripes by eating Limes, or by drinking the Juice. It has likewise been observed, that since the People of Amer-

ica have drank Punch with more Water (which moistens the Feces and dilutes the acrid Salts of the Bile) and made of old Spirit (which has less of the hot fiery Particles than when new from the Still) yet with much more Lime-juice than formerly, the Dry-Gripes is not near so common as before this Custom prevailed (p. 4).

Cadwalader saw rum as the culprit, but also accepted the plethora of other causes listed by his European contemporaries. His remedies were similarly derived from Continental sources. While accepting calomel (mercurous chloride) as a useful therapy for colic, based on his own observations in an autopsy, he rejected the use of quicksilver (elemental mercury). His recommendations were relatively benign.

> The remote Cause is supposed to be an obstructed Perspiration by being to much exposed to a moist Night Air, and cold raw Winds; hard drinking, especially Drams of strong Punch. . . .
> . . . The Method, therefore, to prevent this Malady in such Constitutions is obvious, viz. To abstain, in the West Indies, and in Summer on the Continent, from Drams and strong Punch; salted and high seasoned Meats; immoderate Exercise, which raises Sweat; and profuse Venery (pp. 4–6).

Perhaps of greatest importance, Cadwalader recognized the similarity of the West India dry gripes to industrial lead poisoning. "I have seen in England two Instances of the Success attending the Method here laid down for the Dry-Gripes in the Cholica Pictonum, arising from Fumes of White-lead; which gives Reason to hope, that by a farther Trial of it in Europe, it would be found as beneficial in the latter Distemper, as it is in the former" (p. 28). In 1781, Cadwalader's speculation was proven correct by the chemical detection of lead in Jamaican rum (388).

The significance of Cadwalader's *Essay* has been the subject of considerable debate in the United States (253). On the one hand, it has been acknowledged as one of the earliest contributions to medicine by an American, while on the other, it has been said to lack originality. Cadwalader's description of the dry gripes was essentially similar to earlier reports on the colic of Poitou. The importance of Cadwalader's contribution, however, lies not in the description of symptoms but in his rejection of Citois' theory of acid residues as a cause. He loosened the rigid thinking resulting from traditional European explanations and raised the question of lead. Baker's search for lead in Devonshire cider was, by his own admission, stimulated by his knowledge of the West India dry gripes, transmitted by Benjamin Franklin. Cadwalader's treatise published by Franklin thus deserves recognition as one of the first papers from the American colonies which had significant consequences for medical progress.

This provincial practitioner had an uncommon interest in the etiology of disease and a distaste for theoretical constructions. In the notes for his *Essay* preserved at the College of Physicians of Philadelphia, Calwalader recorded the philosophy which guided his study of the dry gripes. "In all diseases of any kind whatever," he observed in 1717, "it is absolutely necessary to know the cause for otherways it is like a blindman shooting at a mark" (p. 4). He scorned the egotistical professors whose "darling hypothetical systems are but cobweb schemes, rather to show their own parts, than establish a good practice . . . all hypotheses without they are founded on facts."

In a letter to Cadwalader Evans, another colleague at the Pennsylvania Hospital then practicing medicine in Jamaica, Franklin recounted his earlier conversations with Baker on the matter of lead poisoning (252).

> In yours of November 20 [1767] you mention the Lead on the Stills or worms of Stills as a probable cause of the Dry-bellyach among Punch Drinkers in our West India Islands. I had before acquainted Dr. Baker with a Fact of this kind, the general mischief done by the use of Leaden Worms, when Rum Distilling was first practiced in New England, which occasioned a severe Law there against them; and he has mentioned it in the second Part of his piece not yet published. I have long been of the Opinion, that this Distemper proceeds always from a metallic Cause only, observing that its effects among Tradesmen those that use Lead, however different their Trades, as Glazers, Type-Founders, Plumbers, Potters, White Lead-makers and Painters; from the latter, it has been conjectured it took its Name Colica Picton[r]um by the Mistake of a Letter and not from its being the Disease of Poictou, and altho' the Worms of Stills, ought to be of pure Tin, they are often made of Pewter, which has a great Mixture in it of Lead (p. 546).

Franklin's astonishing knowledge of lead paralleled or anticipated that of Europe's finest physicians. Perhaps this was because he lacked a formal medical education. The ghosts of medical tradition seemed to haunt the provincial American scholar less than they did his erudite European counterparts. But Franklin, himself a sufferer from the gout, gave no hint that he suspected lead might be the cause of that affliction, too.

An English physician residing in the West Indies, William Hillary, assisted Franklin in spreading news of the danger of West India rum to Baker. In his *Observations on the Changes in the Air, and the Concomitant Epidemial Diseases in the Island of Barbados* originally published in 1738, Hillary demonstrated his acquaintance with "the Dry Gripes, or Dry Belly-ache endemic to the West Indies" (375).

Sydenham, Cadwalader, and Hillary specifically refer to Riverius as their authority for treating the dry gripes (111, 724). Writing in 1653, Riverius in turn, cited his primary sources, Paul of Aegina and Citois (643). Riverius' therapy of the colic was in the magical tradition and included "the guts of a Wolf in white wine" (592, p. 11). Hillary, fortunately, showed little inclination to follow this prescription, which might have been particularly difficult to fill in Barbados. A more accessible remedy, based on "Horse-Dung" (592, p. 16), recommended by Riverius, was similarly ignored by Hillary. While citing prior sources, Hillary was not bound by their authority. His account of the dry bellyache in Barbados, along with that of Cadwalader, reached George Baker, with historic repercussions.

Just as the ideas of Cadwalader, Hillary, and Franklin were known to Baker, Baker's discoveries were quickly diffused in the American colonies. William Buchan's *Domestic Medicine*, first published in London, in 1772, was promptly reprinted in Philadelphia (103). Packard states this work "was more used than any other book of its kind has been or ever will be" (577, p. 510). Buchan covered the subject of lead colic succinctly (104).

> The *nervous colic* prevails among miners, smelters of lead, plumbers, the manufacturers of white lead &c. It is very common in the cyder counties of England, and is supposed to be occasioned by the leaden vessels used in preparing that liquor. It is likewise a frequent disease in the West Indies, where it is termed "the dry belly-ach" (p. 326).

Buchan recommended the avoidance of "sour fruits, acid and austere liquors" and as benign a treatment as had ever been foisted upon credulous patients. "In the West Indies and on the coast of Guinea, it has been found of great use, for preventing this colic, to wear a piece of flannel around the waist, and to drink an infusion of ginger by way of tea" (p. 327).

In the wake of Baker's reports, William Currie noted that the colica Pictonum had all but disappeared from Philadelphia by 1791 (175).

For these twelve or fifteen years back, I imagined there have not been five persons ill of it in this town, if we except a very few who dealt in lead, and who it was evident derived their disease from that source, such as painters, &c.

This species of Colic was formerly attributed to hard drinking; and it is certain that persons addicted to spiritous liquors were generally the subjects of it; but its rare appearance now cannot be owing to an increase of temperance for I fear it is a melancholy truth, that intemperance is as prevalent at this period as it has been these forty years.

Query? Can this difference be accounted for from the general disuse of pewter? (pp. 24–25).

The colic was nevertheless sufficiently prevalent in the colonies to warrant the attention of patent medicine entrepreneurs. The following advertisement was attached to the back of a theological tract published in 1791 (327): "That excellent Antidote against all Gripings called Aqua anti torminalis, which if taken it not only cures the Gripings of Guts, & Wind Cholick, but preventeth that woful Distemper the Dry Belly Ach. Sold by Benjamin Harris—Price 3s the Half Pint Bottle" (p. 41).

By the time Baker's studies became known in the West Indies, reason born of experiment had lost some of its appeal. Whether because of imprecise chemical methods or the variability of lead in rum, the cause of the dry bellyache became clouded by uncertainty (614).

In 1791, John Bell, writing "On the Use of Ardent Spirits as a Principal Cause of the Mortality Among Soldiers in the West-Indies," observed that the "immediate effect has been ascribed to new rum containing a portion of lead in solution, which is known to be a deleterious poison; this supposition, however, so far as I can judge, appears not to be well founded. Several experiments have been made which have failed to ascertain the presence of lead in new rum" (58, p. 19).

Baker's explanation of the Devonshire colic had been largely forgotten. In 1787 Benjamin Moseley offered his own analysis, "On the Belly-Ache or Colica Pictonum" of the West Indies. Moseley was not only familiar with the works of Citois, Huxham, and Baker but had himself experienced colica Pictonum from Austrian wines (541). But despite his injudicious experience, Moseley specifically rejected Baker's conclusion that lead was the cause of colica Pictonum. Having described the symptoms of lead colic and paresis with considerable accuracy, Moseley attests to cures obtained by drinking of the waters at Bath. With imperturbable confidence he states:

> In habits of body disposed to receive this disease, other diseases will bring it on: so will costivness, astringent medicines, bark, acids, irregularity in diet, check to perspiration, anxiety, and indulging aphrodisiacal passion. . . .
>
> The notion that solutions of lead, from the worms, and other utensils employed in the rum distilleries, are among the common causes of the belly-ache in the West Indies, or that there is ever any detectable quantity of lead in rum, are both equally distant from my opinion, and observations. Such chimeras are the offspring of little chemical, and less medical knowledge (pp. 546–49).

The popularity of strong punch survived the American Revolution. The *American Herbal* of 1801 provided a recipe for "what is called chamber maid's punch," a mixture of lime juice and brandy (705). But a warning was appended: "Some say it is prejudicial to the brain and nervous system; and also, that it generates a colic in some constitutions" (p. 270).

Baker's work also fell into some disrepute in Philadelphia. Describing an epidemic of colica Pictonum arising from apple butter kept in lead-glazed earthenware, William Luckey rejected Baker's explanation. Nevertheless, his editor assured us in a footnote that lead *was* the cause. The symptoms Luckey encountered unnerved him (477).

> The disease made its appearance about the termination of the month of November and beginning of December, 1815; nor did it, as is most commonly the case, make its attack on single and scattered cases, but whole families were subjected to its influence. Whoever has had occasion to witness the ingress of a novel and distressing epidemic can well understand, how difficult it is to convey with the pen any thing like an adequate description of its terrors (p. 501).

But he had more confidence in Moseley than in George Baker.

> You may find, I believe, some remarks on this disease in "Hillary on Barbadoes," which I have not an opportunity of referring to. Sir George Baker has also a paper in the Philosophical Transactions, which I have not seen, although I expect it cannot contain anything uncommon or important, as Mosely speaks of it, without making use of any of his remarks (p. 505).

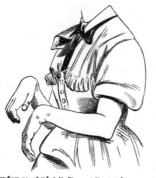

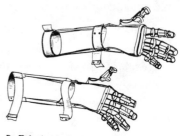

Dr. Hudson's extension apparatus for hands and fingers.

Lead palsy from use of "Laird's Bloom of Youth," from a photograph.

*10. Splint for young ladies whose face powder, Laird's Bloom of Youth,
contained white lead, devised by L. A. Sayre, 1869, professor of orthopedic
surgery at the Bellevue Hospital Medical School (671).*

Siding with the traditionalists, Luckey concluded that repressed perspiration, rather than lead, was the cause.

Despite the credulity of some, America's more astute physicians occasionally identified lead poisoning from both accidental (254, 475) and occupational (206) exposure throughout the nineteenth century. In 1869, Lewis A. Sayre, the first professor of orthopedic surgery of the Bellevue Hospital Medical School, devised an "extension apparatus" (fig. 10), which was constructed by Dr. Hudson (an artificial limb manufacturer) and was reminiscent of Pemberton's earlier device (fig. 4) for the correction of wrist drop. Sayre's patients were fashionable young ladies whose fair complexions were enhanced by both the external and internal effects of a white lead face powder called Laird's Bloom of Youth (671). Innumerable lead-containing cosmetics such as Liebert's Cosmetique Infallible, Eugénie's Favorite, and Ali Ahmed's Treasures of the Desert continued to take their toll among debutantes as the nineteenth century came to a close (75, 560).

"The Most Dreadful Cure"

The possibilities for lead poisoning were by no means limited to rum, cosmetics, and industrial exposure. Although notoriously inefficient as a homicidal agent (737), Christison reports that "in March 1827, a servant-girl was tried for attempting to administer sugar of lead to her mistress in an arrow-root pudding" (145, p. 511). A similar trial of a mother who murdered her infant is recorded by Beck (50). Accidental poisonings were, however, far more common than deliberate ones. In one such tragedy four members of a family of nine died after white lead was accidentally mistaken for sugar. One of the deaths occurred in a nursing infant who absorbed the poison with his mother's milk.

According to some translations of Egyptian medical papyri, medicinal lead was used as early as the second millennium B.C. (311). In his exhaustive review of lead in ancient cultures, Nriagu suggests that Eygptian prescriptions containing lead found their way into the archaic folk medicines of the Mediterranean and Aegean regions (554). Traces of red lead, presumably used for ritual adornment of the deceased, have been found in stone-age burials from about 60,000 B.C. By 6,000 B.C., in pre-Dynastic Egypt, galena was used in eye make-up for the living. In time, the distinction between decoration and function was lost and galena, litharge, and ceruse were included in opthalmic formularies from Greece to China. Although subsequently employed externally for ulcers and wounds throughout the world, early Chinese physicians administered elixirs of lead for the prolongation of life. A paradoxical death was the fate of emperors who sought immortality through alchemical potions (604).

Tanquerel credited Hippocrates with the first use of lead to control uterine hemorrhage. The *Greek Herbal* of Dioscorides offers six prescriptions containing lead but cautions that "burnt lead" is to be removed from the fire only after "having stopped up ye nostrils, for ye vapour is hurtful" (192, p. 631). Rhazes, the ninth-century chronicler of ancient tradition, included lead in his "trochischi albi" (374, p. 23).

Pliny the Elder included litharge mixed with hemlock among medicaments suitable to cure the gout (607, p. 258). The credulous Roman historian also advised lead liniments for the treatment of sores, wounds, hemorrhages, dysentery and as an abortifacient. Ceruse, he noted, "serveth to make an excellent blanche for women, that desire a white complexion; but deadly it is, being taken inwardly in drink" (p. 50). Plates of lead fastened over the kidneys could, Pliny claimed, "coole the heat of fleshly lust" (607).

> And verily Calvus the Orator, who by occasion of much dreaming in sleep of venerous sports, fell into mighty pollutions, and so further into grievous maladie of Gonorrhea or running of the reines with wearing ordinarilly these leaden plates, stayed (by report) all such vaine and wanton fantasies and imaginations; by which means he

preserved also his strength, and had a body able to endure the labor of much study and sitting at his booke (p. 518).

Pliny, nevertheless, knew of the dangers of lead. Manufacturers of paints, he recorded, covered their faces with animal bladders so "that they may take and deliver their wind at libertie, and yet not be in danger of drawing in with their breath that pernicious and deadly powder, which is not better than poyson" (607, p. 477).

The earliest Renaissance texts on metallurgy imply that the use of lead by medieval physicians was commonplace (69). Mercurial ointments soothed the syphilitic sores which plagued Europe following the return of Columbus from the New World. Some claim that these remedies originated with a woman physician of the School of Salerno, Trotula of Salerno (447). Regardless of their origin, it is clear that some of the antisyphilitic ointments contained lead (631, 639). Guy de Chauliac included litharge in his mercurial salve for the treatment of leprosy (311). Agricola described the external application of lead for the treatment of ulcers and to prevent nocturnal emissions in athletes. He attributed these remedies to Galen, failing to acknowledge the influence of his contemporary, Theophrastus Bombastus von Hohenheim, who dubbed himself Paracelsus (7).

Paracelsus introduced lead into the modern pharmacopoeia. Praised as a visionary and denounced as a sorcerer, this peripatetic Swiss physician ushered in the Renaissance for medicine by demanding that observation replace authority. As an alchemist he failed to transmute lead into gold, but did transform it into medicine. "Saturnus purgat febres" (33, p. 332), he claimed. Paracelsus has been credited with first recognizing that kidney stones are a consequence of gout (A1). He had perhaps been influenced by his renowned patient, Desiderius Erasmus, who had declared in 1525 that, "The doctors say that gout and lithiasis are sisters" (A1). Paracelsus treated gout and dropsy with "mercury coagulated with the albumen of eggs" (583, p. 230). Wounds and ulcers he treated with preparations of lead. As much astrologer as physician, Paracelsus had compelling new ideas which suited the intellectual ferment of the Renaissance and were widely disseminated. He held a position somewhere between the alchemists, concerned with mystical significance, and the metallurgists, concerned with practical benefits. With uncompromising arrogance he contested the near sacred tradition of Galenic medicine.

While European critics hounded Theophrastus from city to city, in Britain Paracelsian audacity rode the tide of scientific renewal. Too long mired in humoral theory and received authority, physic stirred to the rumblings of change. Under the influence of Paracelsus, the mystical arts of the alembic began to merge with verifiable experimental endeavor. But the English Paracelsians cloaked scientific innovation in religious orthodoxy (186). In their eyes, Paracelsus was a crusader against the "heathnish and false Philosophie" of Aristotle and Galen. "The Ethnikes doctrines [Aristotelean] standeth upon contemplation, Sophistrie argument, opinion and probabilities of reason without proofs, and commonly fighting against experience" (81, p. 84), wrote R. Bostocke in 1585. In opposition to Galenic theory, Bostocke cited the Hippocratic corpus which, he contended, began with Hermes Trismegistus in ancient Egypt, whose name was an omen of the future coming of the Trinity. The origins of Paracelsian philosophy were found in Christian scripture while, in England, the original "chymicall or spagyrical phylosopher and physician" was identified as Roger Bacon. According to Bostocke, the myth of transmutation of "an Ounce of Quicksilver or Leade into perfect Golde" (p. 46) was but a subterfuge designed to confound would-be abusers of the hermetic arts. Calcination and distillation were the only viable methods for attaining understanding of the "Aetherall Fyre, which nourisheth and quickeneth mans body" (p. 85). "The chymicall physition in his Physicke," he explained, "first and principally respecteth the worde of God, and acknowledgeth it to be his Gifte, next he is ruled by experience" (p. 70).

The evangelical road from alchemy to science had, however, unexpected turns; the route to enlightenment was strewn with conceptual hurdles. Answers to the pithy questions raised by the Paracelsians were not as self-evident as at first surmised. Evolving from the belief in one god and one true religion was the idea of unity in Nature which was in direct opposition to the Galenic doctrine of contraries. Analagous to Adam's fall, every impure thing was deemed to contain within itself the essence of its own cure. "And diseases caused by Quicksilver, Lead or any other thing bee cured by Arcana taken out of them" (p. 76). "So Lead hath in it remedies," observed this chemical philosopher, "for those diseases which be caused and bread in the Miners Leade" (p. 84).

The hermetic arts of ancient Egypt spawned an enduring tradition of polypharmacy and mineral therapies. That tradition, including therapeutic lead, can still be found in the folk medicine of Asia (464), the Middle East (495), and Mexico (2). Health-food faddists are often the modern beneficiaries of these home remedies (169). The prevalence of renal disease among recent Asian immigrants to England has been attributed to the secretive use of a lead-containing aphrodisiac called "rustneg" (20).

Paracelsian fervor was not without its theoretical flights of fancy. Spagyric arts and metaphorical reasoning flourished in the afterglow of intellectual liberation. But rejection of received authority was a necessary step in devising testable hypotheses to examine nature. The fundamental concept of the humors was challenged and, with it, the rationales for purgation, phlebotomy, and polypharmacy. The iconoclastic spirit led to useful insights as well as new therapeutic excesses. In 1651 the chemical philosopher Noah Biggs railed against "the distill'd waters in the leaden stills with peuter-heads" used by apothacaries. Biggs urged the use of glass vessels for such distillations to avoid afflictions of the bowels. In his plea for exploration of the "terra incognita of chemistry" Biggs noted further that similar evils were perpetrated in the home (67).

> Vineger how weak soever, put into a peuter saucer, and suffering it to stand a while, by and by begins to put forth its active, acid corrosive spirit; and in the vineger you shall perceive clearly a certain white mother as it were swimming in the vineger; and the bottome of the saucer, shall be damask'd with white streaks, yea, . . . a certain substance like Cerusse shall be scraped off. . . . This by practice may be observ'd, as by ocular experiment we have try'd, and it is so trivial and common a businesse, that it is known to all Kitchin wenches, but it is not regarded by the most Lady-like stomack (p. 128).

The alchemical philosophers cast a long shadow. Controversy over therapeutic use of metals contributed to the thirty-year delay in publication of the first pharmacopeia in England. The *Pharmacopeia Londinensis* finally appearing in 1618, contained Plumbum Sacharum Saturni (lead acetate), Cerussa (lead carbonate), and Lithargyrum (lead oxide). The Society of Apothecaries, chartered only a year earlier, was quick to embrace Paracelsian innovation (758). Aspirations for magical control over matter passed to chemistry, while the search for eternal life rested uncomfortably at the door of medicine. Expectations of physicians exceeded all reason; their all-too-human failings were but grudgingly tolerated. In the seventeenth and eighteenth centuries this transfer of expectations weighed heavily; the physician's "conjuring book" was written by Hippocrates (fig. 11), his lessons learned at the alchemist's furnace.

With origins emanating from the nether regions of the occult, physicians were never entirely freed of the myth of invincibility. If divine attributes were foisted on some, other practitioners actively cultivated the layman's awe. Faced with almost mystical reverence, they played the god-

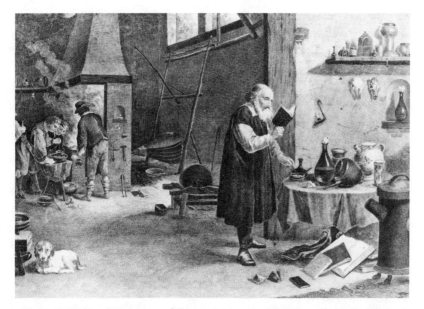

11. Le Grimoire d'Hypocrate *[The conjuring book of Hippocrates], engraved by F. Basam after D. Teniers, about 1780. Medical conjuring was learned at the furnace of the alchemist. From the author's collection.*

like role to the hilt. Paracelsian minerals were blended with Galenic herbs as a practical way of accommodating opposing theories. Salts of lead were gradually added to the witches' brews of plants and animal matter as treatment for virtually all ailments. Gout was included in such therapeutic endeavors (519).

> Sugar of lead may be safely taken inwardly, with appropriate Conserves, and it doth actually mitigate and sweeten (the humors) as its taste doth witness: but it raketh off, and abateth Venerial desires (perhaps much to the advantage of the Gouty Patient.) These sort of Medicines ought to be exhibited in Wain of the Moon, having before made use of the gentler kind of Eccoprotick, or easie purging Medicines (p. 51).

Such therapeutic innovation encouraged quackery. London's most celebrated seventeenth-century "Quack-Astrologer" (747) and self-proclaimed "Professor of Physic," William Salmon, treated "colic due to circumvolution of the Intestines through a Wind" with "leaden or golden Bullets, swallowed down" (666, p. 706). "If the Cholick tends to, or ends in a Palsy," Salmon recommended three doses of horse-dung mixed with poppy water and vitriol.

Enthusiasm for minerals as therapeutic agents met with some resistance. The great English naturalist and colleague of Hooke, Newton, and Boyle, Nehemiah Grew, recorded lead ores among the young Royal Society's early collections of natural "rarities." In his 1674 catalogue of specimens which were to become the foundation of the British Museum, he noted of preparations of lead that, "Many bold Chymists, without Discretion, give inwardly and also extol them. But those that are careful of their Health, will beware of them" (333, p. 330). Yet, in 1751, John Hill did "affirm with great Certainty that it [sugar of lead] will succeed when nothing else is of Effect in Hemorrhages" (374, p. 24).

The leading Dutch physician of the eighteenth century, Herman Boerhaave, furthered the cause of medicinal lead (284). In 1709, Boerhaave advised the use of lead and mercury for the treatment of scirrous cancers (722). Bridging the gap between alchemy and chemistry, Boerhaave reproduced many of the chemical reactions described in spagyric writings. He could not dismiss even the most mystical offerings without a trial. He redistilled lead in his private laboratory for twenty years in the vain hope of achieving transmutation (471). Boerhaave counted among his students the most influential men of European medicine including Haller, Cullen, Pringle, Hillary, Huxham, de Haen, Tronchin, van Swieten, and Von Storck. Prescriptions for heavy metals were gradually extended to epilepsy, dropsy, and hemorrhage—therapeutic modalities which found strong professional support for two centuries (678).

Despite the controversial nature of medicinal lead, *The New Dispensatory* of 1753 instructed pharmacists in the ways of making a variety of saturnine preparations. It advises that the sugar of lead is particularly efficacious but warns, "it occasions symptoms of another kind, often more dangerous than those removed by it, and sometimes fatal" (459, p. 325). Similar contradictory advice was given by Robert James in *The Modern Practice of Physic* of 1746 (397).

George Baker uncompromisingly opposed the medicinal use of lead (31). "Yet surely," he warned, "physicians cannot be too cautious in avoiding the use of medicines, the effect of which, for aught they can presume to ascertain, may be more formidable then the very disease to which they are opposed" (p. 236).

Learning the lessons of the Devonshire colic was slow and often painful in Europe as well as in the colonies. For every stride forward there was a step backward. Toward the end of the eighteenth century Goulard's secret "extract of saturn" attained singular popularity (316). "This liquor," proclaimed Goulard, "may very well be substituted in the place of wine and brandy (in every case where these are generally used), as likewise in that of different embrocations, commonly prescribed for inflammation" (p. 6). The therapeutic benefits of his diacetate of lead were, he professed, distinct from the harmful effects of lead acetate (316).

> The comparison made between extract of Saturn and its salt, commonly called the sugar of lead, will be found unjust, when we consider that the latter is made with vinegar of all sorts of wine. . . . A practice of fifty years has sufficienty convinced me of its superiority over the sugar of lead, which I have known fail, when the other has always answered my intentions. . . . The Extract of Saturn is also efficacious in periodical pains that attack the joints, and are termed gouty (p. 117).

Goulard's "vegeto-mineral waters" were recommended primarily for external use: absorption of lead was minimized if patients followed the explicit rather than implicit instructions. Absorption through mucous membranes or denuded surfaces such as burns was nevertheless possible. George Baker reported several cases of severe lead poisoning due to Goulard's extract, even when applied externally (32, 36). It was, however, widely believed that if external application was good, internal use could only be better. This misconception was fostered by Goulard's efforts to reap financial benefit from his fashionable remedy. In Britain, he authorized George Arnaud de Ronsil, "doctor in physic in the University of Tubingen," to be the sole distributor of the authentic extract (18). Arnaud touted the Water of Saturn, with equal enthusiasm, for the treatment of horses and of the gout.

In his *Cautions to the Heads of Families*, John Fothergill, the distinguished English physician and benefactor of the first American medical school in Philadelphia, supported the medicinal use of lead (267). Fothergill was, nevertheless, well aware of its dangers. In 1776, he reported to the Society of Physicians in London a number of unusual ways in which lead intoxication might be acquired including watercolor paints, medicines, and childhood pica (266). Fothergill advised his readers that the colics of Poitou, Devonshire, and the West Indies all had the same origin and cited English wine-making as a particularly insidious source of lead poisoning.

The antidiarrheal properties of lead were widely expoited. Alderson informs us that (13):

> De Haen mentions a case in which a scruple of the acetate, and a drachm of the carbonate, were given together in six ounces of water, to be taken by teaspoonfuls. Soon after taking some of it, the patient was seized with excruciating pain in the bowels, followed by vomiting, and seems narrowly to have escaped with life; while it is stated that for three years afterwards he had reason to lament "the lingering remains of that most dreadful cure." At the present time lead in the form of acetate is still in good reports for the cure of a certain class of diseases, the same for which Celsus recommended the "plumbnum combustum" (p. 96).

American military physicians were reluctant to relinquish lead acetate prescriptions. In his *Medical Sketches*, James Mann, an American army surgeon during the War of 1812, reported that the indiscriminant use of lead acetate to treat diarrhea among the troops was responsible for a rash of "dropsical swellings" (510, p. 131). Mann understood the dropsy in the conventional terms of his times: "translation of the disease." "The checking of a diseased secretion of one organ," he wrote, "may induce a diseased action of another" (511, p. 19). Dropsy was thus an expected consequence of effective therapy of colica Pictonum. He had no way of suspecting lead nephropathy, heart disease, or acute tubular necrosis (from therapeutic mercury) as possible causes of fluid retention.

Deaths from medicinal lead occurred among officers as well as enlisted men (511). Adulterated rum was, apparently, so familiar to this military surgeon, that it was among his first thoughts when he encountered a case of lead poisoning. In 1822 he began a report in the *New England Journal of Medicine* as follows:

> A disease marked with all the symptoms of Colica Pictonum has a conspicuous place on my sick report for the month of August last: The unusual number attacked with this formidable complaint, induced suspicions, that there "was death in the pot." Upon strict examination, it was ascertained, the disease did not originate from kitchen utensils. Liquors drunk by the men were also suspected to have been adulterated with acetite of lead; these were tested, without giving the usual evidence of the existence of a mineral poison (p. 17).

It is no wonder that physicians and laymen alike were confused about the therapeutic value of lead. Compounds of the metal were advocated in many quarters. Although John Wesley was aware of lead colic, the recipes added to his *Primitive Physic*, a century after its initial publication, contained the following remedies (802):

> Vinegar of Litharge. Take of litharge, half a pound; strong vinegar, two pints. Infuse them together, in a moderate heat, for three days, frequently shaking the vessel; then filter the liquor for use.
>
> This medicine is in little used from a general notion of its being dangerous. There is reason, however, to believe that the preparations of lead with vinegar are possessed of some valuable properties, and that they may be used in many cases with safety and success (p. 128).

Heated debate about the therapeutic value of lead continued well into the nineteenth century (700). Lead acetate was not only widely used to check diarrhea including that associated with terminal uremia (144, 331) but was held by many to be an unsurpassed remedy for internal bleeding (678). In 1905, British physicians still found it necessary to alert the public to the tragic consequences resulting from lead compounds taken for "female irregularities" and to induce abortions (346). Nor has lead been entirely purged from modern clinical practice (87, 324). As recently as 1925, lead was given intravenously for the treatment of cancer (59), a mode of administration that induces a devastating form of renal disease—acute tubular necrosis—not encountered after oral administration. Acute tubular necrosis is potentially fatal. It has, however, rarely been encountered from lead in recent times except following the accidental introduction of lead acetate into a vein by drug abusers (49, 215).

In America, lead found its way into the prescriptions of the most proper of Bostonians. James Thacher, the first historian of American medicine, preserved ancient therapeutic traditions along with his accounts of emerging scholarship in the new nation. In his *American Modern Practice* of 1817, the "approved formula applicable to the diseases of our climate" (741) included "Saturnine Anodyne Pills," which were thought to be particularly efficacious in uterine hemorrhage.

Although lead poisoning from rum appeared to have declined considerably in Philadelphia, colica Pictonum was still to be found among lead workers. Describing his ministrations to employees of a white lead plant in 1820, Dr. Richard Harlan devised a remedy in the true Paracelsian tradition. After mercury and opium failed he "found no remedy so well adapted to the purpose, as sugar of lead" (355, p. 21). Harlan attributed this therapeutic revelation to his observations of the efficacy of saccharum saturni in cases of dysentery. "Four cases only" he admitted, "have terminated fatally under my own treatment." Three of these he attributed to "habitual drunkenness" (p. 22), and the other was "an ignorant German" who delayed too long in seeking treatment.

The conflicting opinions about medicinal lead presented no small dilemma to practicing physicians. Information "generally received" was notoriously vague with respect to dosage. Even the most diligent practitioner could find no reliable data on proper quantities and was forced to determine dosage by trial and error. Uncontrolled trials invariably substantiated wishful thinking.

Faced with the "formidable array, before me, the phanthoms, paralysis, convulsions, colica, and perhaps even death . . . of those whose health and safety we are engaged and bound to preserve to the utmost of our skill" (p. 149), the surgeon William Laidlaw tested lead acetate on himself in order to ascertain the safe dose (434). Laidlaw concluded that ten grains a day for five days was the upper limit of tolerance since he did not develop colic on this regimen until the sixth day. With impressive sincerity but faulty information, he proceeded to treat his patients according to his finding. Laidlaw substituted good intentions for the scientific method. He did not report the results of his therapy.

The risk of poisoning from therapeutic excess was compounded by the risk of accidental contamination of medicine. Vivum (wine) and brandy, cornerstones of the early pharmacopoeia, were hailed by some as wholesome stimulants to appetite and spirit. But others held a more gloomy view. "Nature resents the injury in the form of gout, palsy and apoplexy" (780, p. 18), Benjamin Waterhouse cautioned his medical students in 1804. His moral outrage may have had a toxicologic basis since the danger of adulteration of medicinal preparations was no less than that of beverages. In 1846, Lewis C. Beck, professor of chemistry at Rutgers, published qualitative analytic methods for the detection of lead in substances listed in the *United States Pharmacopoeia*. At the same time, Beck described methods for detecting lime and iron contaminating medicinal lead acetate (50). Pharmaceutical manufacturers did not always consider consumer protection the top priority.

The side effects of medicinal lead suited the satirist's prescription for

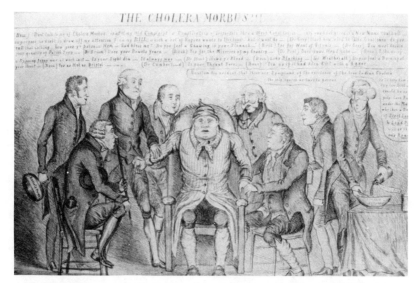

12. The treatment for The Cholera Morbus !!! *was "lead pills," about 1835.*
From the collection of William Helfand.

politicians. Political ills required harsh treatment. For John Bull's cholera
morbus, one cartoonist proclaimed that "*Steel Lozenges & Lead Pills* will
be the only *Remedy*" (fig. 12).

Commercial Zeal

Therapeutic use of lead encouraged a callous attitude in the industrial
setting where protective measures were virtually nonexistent. The industrial revolution evolved with little concern for the health of workers. Use
of lead skyrocketed and artisans fortunate enough to find employment
considered industrial hazards the legitimate price for work. The Diderot
Encyclopedia illustrates a furnace hood funneling away the scorching
heat from an eighteenth-century lead smelter (fig. 13). No such protection diverted the fumes over the open troughs in which the molten metal
solidified. Along the manufacturing chain, other artisans suffered similar
hazards as the sheets of lead were processed into water pipes, pewter,
paint, and other commercial products.

Appreciation of the danger to lead workers emerged slowly. In 1678,
Vernatti expanded Stockhausen's 1656 description of the sufferings of
lead miners to include occupations involved in the manufacturing of lead

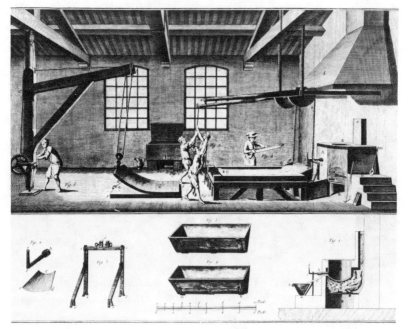

13. Lead foundry, engraving from Laminage du plomb *in the* Diderot
Encyclopedia, *1780.*

products. He noted that lead dust and "steams" were responsible for
anorexia, vomiting, constipation, colic, blindness, and "stupidity" (764).
Soon thereafter, Antony van Leeuwenhoek warned the members of the
Royal Society that potters, too, were subject to lead poisoning. In 1685,
Leeuwenhoek published in the *Philosophical Transactions* the first illustrations of crystals of calcined lead as they appeared in the microscope
(fig. 14, [451]).

> Our Porcellan Bakers use much Tin, or Lead, which they calcine
> in their Ovens. This work . . . is so prejudicall to those that tend it,
> that a man can't stand before the mouth of the Oven, above 24
> hours at a time, and then he looks as if he was poysoned; so that
> every day a fresh man is employed to take care of the Oven, and
> remove the scum from the surface of the Lead (p. 1082).

Manufacturers were quick to perceive that it was more profitable to ro-
tate the workers than to provide ventilation. Rotation of workers remains
a main line of defense in the contemporary lead industry (755).

Transmitted knowledge, supported by myth and common experience,

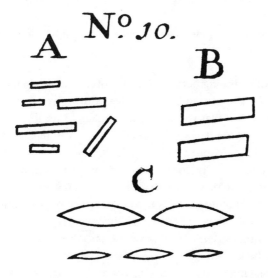

14. *Crystals of calcined lead as seen by Antony van Leeuwenhoek,*
1685 (451).

proved to be an unreliable teacher. Eyewitnesses testified to the procrea-
tion of metals within the earth, the womb which nurtured metalic seeds
to perfection. Those privy to this truth were not easily dissuaded. Theirs
was a secret demonstrable in every day's experience. Authorities from
Aristotle to Boyle cited the breeding and growth of metals in underground crypts. Under auspicious circumstances, the most imperfect of
metals would "ripen, . . . from one degree of perfection to another, as
from Lead to Silver" (785, p. 71). In 1671, John Webster credited Galen
and Agricola with the observation "that Lead being placed in a moist cel-
lar or subterranean rooms, where the air is gross and turbid, will be increased in both bulk and weight" (785, p. 70). The spontaneous generation of metals linked chemistry to alchemy even as verifiable hypotheses
began to replace mystical conjecture and ancient teachings were subject
to rigorous reexamination.

As the seventeenth century drew to a close, Nicholas Lemery summarized the more sophisticated views of the chemistry of lead (455).

Lead is a Metal filled with Sulphurs, or a Bitumous earth, that renders it very Supple and Pliant. It is probable that it contains some
Mercury. It hath pores very like those of Tinn; it is called Saturn by

the reason of the influence it is thought to receive from the Planet of that name.

Those who work upon Lead are subject to Colicks and become Paralytick (p. 105).

Lemery's understanding of the chemistry of lead embodied the state of the art. He noted the gain in weight of lead during calcination—a conceptual contradiction that would not be explained until a century later by Lavoisier. The "volatile parts of Lead do fly away in Calcination," he observed, "which loss should indeed make it weigh the less, nevertheless after a long Calcination 'tis found that instead of losing, it increases in weight." Rejecting the possibility that the increased weight derived from the coal, Lemery concluded, " 'Tis better therefore to refer this effect to the disposition of the Pores of Lead in such a manner, that part of the fire insinuating into them does there remain embodied, and can't get forth again, whence the weight comes to be encreased" (p. 107). And with this reasonably satisfying explanation consistent with traditional concepts of the four elements, the matter rested. The question, rephrased, eroded the phlogiston theory a century later and begged for new answers. While not the first to note that calcined metals gained rather than lost weight, Lemery demystified the observation.

No mention of lead was made in the first modern textbook of toxicology by Richard Mead in 1702. In the third edition, published in 1745, a single paragraph sufficed to warn readers that lead could be an occupational hazard. Compared to the more dramatic and deadly effects of snake bites, arsenic, or mercury, lead was seen as relatively inconsequential (523).

The full extent of occupational exposure to lead was still only vaguely perceived when Bernardino Ramazzini published the first comprehensive text on *Diseases of Workers* in 1700 (620). While professor of the practice of medicine at Padua, Ramazzini exerted a crucial influence on his younger colleague, Morgagni, who was to become the founder of modern pathologic anatomy. The idea, nurtured by these men, that diseases could be classified in accordance with observable causes was to mold the course of medicine. The impact of Ramazzini's description of occupational diseases was comparable to that of Morgagni's seminal descriptions of pathology. By 1714, Ramazzini could list over ten occupations at which workers "habitually incur serious maladies from the deadly fumes of metals"—goldsmiths, alchemists, distillers of aqua fortis (nitric acid), potters, mirror makers, founders, tinsmiths, painters, smelters, and chemists. Since occupational exposure usually included a myriad of metallic vapors, Ramazzini did not distinguish lead toxicity from that of mercury, antimony, cadmium, copper, or arsenic.

Following directly in the experimental tradition of alchemy, chemistry, too, subjected its adherents to poisoning from metallic fumes. "We must not laugh at a chemist," warned Ramazzini, "if he sometimes comes out of his laboratory looking haggard and dogged as though he belonged to the gods of the underworld."

One wonders if Ramazzini had Isaac Newton in mind. The rationality of the great seventeenth-century physicist was well known to be fragile. Newton's "derangement of intellect" of 1693 has recently been ascribed to mercury poisoning following analysis of hair reputed to be his (217, 696). The paucity of supporting evidence of mercurialism has prompted some psychiatrists to propose a diagnosis of hereditary manic depression (462). From the data presented, Newton's insomnia, paranoia, and seclusiveness might just as readily have been attributed to lead. Newton pursued alchemical experiments with compulsive intensity over several decades yet never displayed the characteristic tremor of mercurialism. Rather, his bizarre behavior was followed by the gout, a complication of plumbism. The amount of lead Newton absorbed during his alchemical studies is a secret which may yet reside with his bones in Westminster Abbey. Resolution of the question may still be feasible since the diagnosis of lead poisoning has been established retrospectively by analysis of bone in other famous men, for example, Pope Clemens II (d. 1046, [697]), and the ill-fated sons of Ivan the Terrible (d. sixteenth century, [322]).

Only in the case of potters was Ramazzini specific in naming lead as the cause of pallor, cachexia, and palsy. To these workmen he recommended removal from exposure, assiduous cleanliness, and iron therapy. But Ramazzini's sources were largely received authority and contemporary anecdotes. He included among etiologic considerations the "little demons and phantoms" (p. 26), which, according to Agricola, haunted the underground passages and wrought havoc among miners. The transition from alchemy to science was not yet complete and the devil was still believed to have a tight grip on nature.

The earliest evidence of industrial production of lead in England is an ingot dated just seven years after the Roman occupation, A.D. 49 (315). Although the refined metal was probably destined for export to Rome, local use in water pipes and pewter at the time has recently been documented (322). Specimens have been found from 1500 B.C. in Egypt, but pewter plates, tankards, bowls, and spoons first achieved widespread popularity in Roman Britain (554). Kitchen utensils were commonly half lead, half tin. There is reason to believe that the mining of lead in Britain preceded Roman subjugation and was ripe for exploitation at the time of the Roman conquest. Records of the industrial hazards are, however, conspicuously lacking until the seventeenth century, when the Royal Society, at the behest of Robert Boyle, recorded current mining techniques and, in passing, noted the dangers inherent to smelters (315). The concern of the society was, however, with commercial development rather than with the health of the workman.

A detailed description of industrial lead poisoning appeared in *Scotts Magazine* in 1754. Workers at the Leadhill mine were subject to what was commonly called "mill reek": severe attacks of colic and encephalopathy often followed by palsies (524, 812). In the same year *Scotts Magazine* published James Lind's tentative speculation that the abdominal complaints attributed to lemon juice were probably caused by lead leached from ceramic earthenware. Lind achieved medical immortality by proving that lemon juice could prevent scurvy among British seamen. This remedy proved so effective that it was also soon used in the treatment of colic.

Tinned copper pots were no safer than glazed earthenware. Their silvery coats, achieved with the liberal application of lead, gave luster to kitchenware and assurance that copper would not be leached into the foods they contained. In 1756, the Society for the Encouragement of Art, Manufacturers and Commerce offered a prize to anyone who could devise a method of "tinning" that did not require lead, but there were no takers (810). Responsibility for prevention of lead poisoning in the home rested with no institution and there was no profit in it.

Protection of workmen had no place in the agenda of the pioneers of industry. Occupational safety conflicted with aspirations for the wealth of the nation. In the eighteenth century, the orphanages of London were emptied by apprenticing the children to cotton mills. Eight-year-olds labored for fourteen hours a day under appalling conditions. Steeped in filth and stunted by malnutrition, the paupers were plagued by consumption, rickets, and epidemic infections. Only as the steam engine reduced the need for unskilled labor and tuberculosis threatened the entire community, did pity appear to ameliorate commercial zeal. Sir Robert Peel, a millowner himself, won the first government action to alleviate the conditions of the mill children, the Health and Morals Act of 1802 (244). The act proclaimed that the children should not work more than twelve hours a day, nor sleep more than two to a bed, and should be taught to read. But since provision for enforcement was omitted, working conditions in the cotton mills did not change.

The glimmerings of reform that flickered in the cotton mills shifted to the potteries where the social cost of exploitation was compounded by the noxious fumes of lead. With the introduction of glazed earthenware of 1670, Staffordshire became the center for pottery manufacturing in England (137). In 1816, Josiah Wedgewood, a sometime scientist and leading manufacturer, deplored the danger of glazes and pressed for improvements in the factories (244). At Wedgewood's behest, efforts were begun to devise glazes with reduced quantities of soluble lead.

In an 1831 treatise on occupational medicine, Charles Turner Thackrah listed the professions subject to lead poisoning: miners, ironworkers, founders, brass workers, solderers, and potters. Of workmen around Leeds he reports (744): "Smelting is considered a most fatal occupation. The appearance of the men is haggard in the extreme." Of plumbers: "The occupation undermines the constitution, for plumbers are short lived. I learn that there are but two individuals in Leeds and the neighborhood, who have regularly pursued this employ beyond the age of 40" (p. 81). Of painters: "Painters are unhealthy in appearance, and do not generally attain full age. Their maladies are evidently the result of an impression on the nervous system, through the medium of the membranes of the nostrils and the air tube. The more serious permanent evils of working in paint are colic and palsy" (p. 82).

In 1837 the Medical Society of New York awarded a prize of $50 for an essay by Benjamin McCready on "The influence of trades, professions and occupations in the United States in the production of disease." McCready recorded the occurrence of colica Pictonum and wrist drop among typesetters and painters in the New York area. He also cited cases of insanity due to lead encountered in the New York Lunatic Asylum (489). Among miners, the consequences of lead poisoning were obscured by the overwhelming pulmonary disease that accompanied that occupation (246). The potteries remained the most dramatic setting for observing lead poisoning.

Ineffective as the act of 1802 was, it established the responsibility of government for the health and welfare of industrial workers. Despite repeated investigations and new factory acts, by 1851 five thousand boys and girls, five to fifteen years of age still worked in the Staffordshire potteries, twelve to fifteen hours a day, six days a week (137). Testimony before the Childrens Employment Commission in 1862 revealed "that paralysis, colica Pictonum, epilepsy and a host of nervous diseases, are to be met with in all their aggravated forms" (p. xxvi). But the evidence indicated that progress had been made. According to one child, " 'tis not so bad now as formerly, when a greater proportion of the poisonous metal entered into the composition of the liquid [glaze]" (p. xxv). "Should a remedy be suggested," one witness testified, "the children would have reason to hail the day of their emancipation from the toil little removed from slavery" (p. xxvii). The commission proposed to achieve this goal by requiring a Certificate of Education attesting to the ability of the apprentices to read the Testament before they reached the age of fifteen.

For a time, the plight of women captured the public imagination. The frequent miscarriages and birth defects were dealt with by refusing women employment. In 1876, the minimum working age was raised to ten years and rules were promulgated by the British government to provide minimum sanitation. In 1892, pottery manufacturing was deemed a dangerous trade and in 1894 the minimum employment age was raised to fourteen.

Opposition to government regulation was relentless. Incomplete epidemiologic data was an easy target for obfuscation by professional spokesmen for the lead industry. Pleading economic hardship, employers asserted that the problem was greatly exaggerated, the data inadequate and that poisoning, if it occurred, was the result of carelessness on the part of the workmen. Plumbism, they claimed, was in fact due to arsenic. The adversary stance resulted in perennially shifting government policy. Progress was retarded but not stopped. The responsibility was established, and in 1898, Thomas Legge was appointed the first Medical Inspector of Factories. Glazes containing minimal amounts of low-solubility lead were required throughout the pottery industry and high-lead glazes prohibited. Of most importance, by 1903, the consequences of industrial lead poisoning came under compulsory compensation. Financial incentives were thereby created to encourage plant owners to provide a safe workplace.

These achievements in industrial health took over a century to accomplish, but the battle lines remained fixed. Safety, initially defined in terms of preventing overt symptoms and death, has been extended to include the monitoring of blood lead levels. But the more subtle delayed effects of chronic low-level absorption have yet to be eliminated. Confusion, speculation, and polemics will continue to prevent corrective action as long as objective methods for detecting low-level absorption remain in doubt.

But even overt symptoms go unnoticed by physicians lacking motivation to recognize disease among the laboring classes. In Derbyshire, for
example, doctors were unimpressed by the symptoms exhibited by the
local galena miners. In 1857, Dr. William Webb extolled the "picturesque
and highly salubrius" surroundings of the mineral district of South Derbyshire (784). "It consists," Webb observed, "principally of hill and dale,
and of natural scenery which, for grandeur and beauty, it would be difficult if not impossible to surpass" (p. 687). These idyllic surroundings
combined with frequent outdoor exercise, short work hours, personal
cleanliness, and good food were responsible for the miners' remarkable
"health and longevity." The pallor and prostration they demonstrated
Webb attributed to the lack of oxygen in the mines. Their colic, paresis,
blue-line of the gums, rheumatism responsive to colchicine, fatal falls,
lung diseases, and injuries from explosives he accepted as accidents that
necessarily accompanied such work.

The gentry were sometimes more empathetic to the plight of animals.
The toxic effluvia of industry played havoc with beasts beyond the con-
fines of the factories. Although concern for the fate of lead workers did
not reach official records until the nineteenth century, the economic
threat of industrial pollution to domestic cattle was the subject of duly
recorded legal proceedings (315). In sixteenth-century Britain the smelters presented an unwelcome incursion into the agrarian society. Water,
used to wash the crude ore, and smoke, emanating from the smelters, carried deadly particles to the neighboring fields and streams. Fish disappeared from the lakes where wildlife had previously abounded. "I know a
small rivulet, on which some of these mills stand, wherein trouts have
been caught . . ." wrote Dr. John Carte, "their heads being great and mis-
shapen, their backs crooked, their tails very small, which I am apt to believe might proceed from them feeding on the smithram or dust" (598,
p. 462).

Modern environmentalists have pursued their goals with mounting
vigor. Fish have returned to the Thames. But in pursuit of the renewed
aquatic life have come fishermen, with lead-weighted sinkers (544). The
royal swans, impervious to industrial pollutants of the past, are succumb-
ing to the lead weights. To their peril, the swans mistake the sinkers for
food and the clean-up of the Thames has devastated the queen's stately
birds.

But in the seventeenth century, industrial pollution was just gaining
momentum. Sheep, cattle, and dogs lapping water contaminated by the

refining operations were seen to whirl in endless circles followed by a frightening lethargy just before expiring (563, 597). Dogs and cats "often kill themselves by running headlong into a wall" (597, p. 23). Domestic animals afflicted with cerebral plumbism were called "bellond," a traditional term for painter's colic in Derbyshire (861, 784). Robert James reported that "a certain Space round the Smelting-houses is called Bellon ground, where it is dangerous for any animal to feed" (396). Deer roaming the forests in the vicinity of the smelters displayed bizarre deformities of their antlers and this, too, was attributed to the smoke settling across the countryside.

In 1981, a similar episode was noted in northwestern Louisiana. A farmer reported that twenty of his cows had circled aimlessly for a few minutes, then sat down and expired. These deaths were the result of lead paint from a nearby sandblasted bridge which had contaminated their forage (245).

In 1861 Charles Dickens captured the persisting plight of the poor, forced to seek employment in the white-lead works (188).

> The borders of Ratcliff and Stepney, eastward of London, and giving on the impure river, were the scene of this uncompromising dance of death, upon a drizzling November day. A squalid maze of streets, courts, and alleys of miserable houses let out in hunger. A mud-desert, chiefly inhabited by a tribe from whom employment has departed or to whom it comes but fitfully and rarely. . . .
>
> I saw a horrible brown heap on the floor in the corner, which, but for previous experience in this dismal wise, I might not have suspected to be "the bed". There was something thrown upon it; and I asked what that was.
>
> "'Tis the poor craythur that stays here, sur; and 'tis very bad she is, and 'tis very bad she's been this long time, and 'tis better she'll never be, and 'tis slape she does all day, and 'tis wake she does all night, and 'tis the lead, sur."
>
> "The what?"
>
> "The lead, sur. Sur 'tis the lead mills, where the women gets took on at eighteen-pence a day, sur, when they makes application early enough, and is lucky and wanted; and 'tis lead pisoned she is, sur, and some of them gets lead-pisoned soon and some of them gets lead-pisoned later, and some, but not many, niver; and 'tis all according to the constitooshun, sur, and some constitooshuns is strong, and some is weak; and her constitooshun is lead-pisoned,

bad as can be, sur; and her brain is coming out at her ear, and it hurts her dreadful; and that's what it is, and niver no more, and niver no less, sur" (pp. 289–91).

Women were preferentially employed in the manufacture of paint since they were reputed to be less susceptible than men to the malignant influence of the white powder. The high turnover of young female employees was attributed to their dissolute ways until Thomas Oliver suggested that women were, in fact, more susceptible than men to lead. Menstrual abnormalities and spontaneous abortions were their lot soon after exposure (562). Oliver reported that lead poisoning could be transferred in utero and described lead-induced interstitial nephritis in the newborn infant of a white-lead worker. He also noted that abnormalities in the sperm of male workers were associated with infertility and fetal malformations.

No occupation was more subject to lead poisoning than the production of white lead for paint. As early as 1775, the French chemist Guyton de Morveau had advised the elimination of lead-based paints and the substitution of zinc paints as a public health measure (563). In 1852, a Special Committee of the Board of Assistant Aldermen of New York City recommended that lead-based paint be replaced with "zinc paint on property of the city, both on account of its superior healthfulness, and greater economy" (76, p. 2). Had this committee's advice been taken for private as well as city property, New York's pica crisis, a century later, would not have occurred. In England, legislation to control white-lead plants was finally enacted in 1892 (736). Enforcement was, however, less than rigorous since, in 1898, thirty-seven white-lead workers under eighteen years of age died of plumbism in these paint factories (563).

In the United States, lead in interior house paints came under federal regulation by the Consumer Product Safety Commission in 1976, but exterior paint is still beyond the control of federal law. Interior paint must contain less than 60 mg of lead per gm dry paint while the lead content of exterior paint is left to the discretion of the manufacturer and local ordinance.

Industrial lead poisoning had been common in the United States until the early part of the present century. Even then, physicians of the young nation were readily assured by the captains of industry that all was well in the workplace. The works of Daniel Drake, pioneer of medicine west of the Mississippi, reflected the complacency of the industrial revolution and the limitations imposed by diagnostic methodology (199).

Several years ago, when smelting was performed in rude log fur-
naces, colic was common but, since the introduction of those of a
better construction, which carry off the fumes, it has become rare.
In visiting one of the best, I perceived a peculiar taste in the air; but
its proprietor assured me that none of his operators ever experience attacks of colic or paralysis (p. 694).

It was generally believed that when lead poisoning occurred it was the
fault of the workman. Serene optimism was reflected in the American
Public Health Association prize essay of 1886. Citing the case of a painter
who developed symptoms of plumbism, the winner attributed the mis-
fortune to the victim's "gossiping nature" (p. 18). He considered talking
at work dangerous because it causes increased breathing through the
nose (393). Silence was the best protection for lead workers.

Despite such assurances, a 40 percent incidence of symptomatic lead
intoxication was found (357) at a time when occupational health standards were virtually nonexistent. Writing of working conditions in 1910,
the pioneering American industrial health physician Alice Hamilton observed that "employers could, if they wished, shut their eyes to the dangers their workmen faced, for nobody held them responsible, while the
workers accepted the risks with fatalistic submissiveness as part of the
price one must pay for being poor" (349, p. 4). There was neither the will
nor the data to promote occupational safety.

Impressive as were the scientific advances during the first part of the
twentieth century, some were, at times, misleading. "The earliest symptom of lead poisoning," insisted Thomas Legge, "is anemia" (453, p. 28),
implying that without anemia symptoms could not be attributed to lead.
The experts further advised that continuous exposure induces "tolerance" to lead (p. 29). If symptoms persisted, the worker was deemed pe-
culiarly susceptible and removed from his job.

Physicians were advised that lead nephropathy could not occur in the
absence of overt symptoms of lead intoxication such as colic, palsy, or
encephalopathy. "There is no experimental evidence," declared one expert in 1925 of the Broken Hill Mine in Australia, "that exposure to doses
of lead, insufficient to cause classical signs of lead poisoning, will cause
tissue damage to the arteries and the kidneys" (690, p. 393). Retrospective examination of mortality data at this mine has recently proven
this assertion to be false (493).

Since the beginning of this century the severity of lead exposure in
American industry has been greatly curtailed. Symptomatic plumbism is

rarely encountered now (640) and new diagnostic techniques capable of uncovering dangerous body lead stores in the absence of symptoms make it possible to detect organ damage before overt plumbism occurs. The new tools have not, however, been exploited. The forces which delay the application of medical knowledge are similar today to those of the past. Industry has recently favored reliance on measurement of blood lead for monitoring plant safety. As long as the employee's blood lead remained within federal guidelines, the employer was protected whether or not employees became ill. In-depth research on occupational lead exposure was virtually nonexistent.

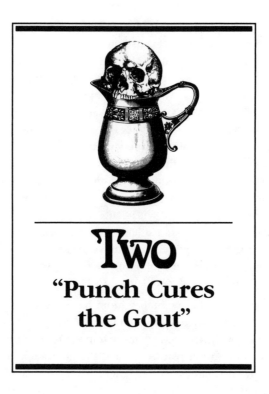

Two

"Punch Cures the Gout"

Of Bacchus and Venus

While alcoholic drinks were occasionally credited with causing the colic followed by the palsy, the indictment of wine as a cause of gout was universal. For almost two millennia, this etiologic concept achieved unquestioning acceptance and then gradually faded away. Contradictory experience throughout the world undermined confidence in the causal relationship (668) which seems to have been more forgotten than systematically excluded. It has recently been suggested that the association of port wine with gout was coincidental; the wine merely washed down those epicurean repasts which the body converts to uric acid (363). Another explanation for the gradual change in medical thinking is that it was not the wine but an inconstant contaminant of wine which predisposed to gout. Because this contaminant is absent from most modern wines, the association has been lost. The long and colorful history of gout suggests that one key variable may have been lead.

The earliest descriptions of lead poisoning gave no hint that gout might be a complication (775). Vitruvius warned that mineral springs arising near mines might promote the gout (554), but, in accord with Hippocrates, gout was regarded primarily as an hereditary disease of middle-aged men. As Rome wallowed in opulence, however, gout became increasingly linked with drunkenness and gluttony (555). A change in the pattern of the afflication soon became apparent. The Romans found gout occurring with increasing frequency among women. "The nature of women has not altered but their manner of living," wrote Seneca, "for while they rival men in every kind of licentiousness, they equal them too in their bodily disorders. Why need we then to be suprised at seeing so many of the female sex afflicted with gout?" (320, p. 486).

This change in clinical picture, also noted by Galen (399), was of considerable interest in eighteenth-century London where the disease reached epidemic proportions. John Rotheram, in a footnote to his 1793 translation of Cullen's works, proclaimed (172):

> Hippocrates says that women seldom have the gout and never before the disappearance of the catamenia [menses]. In his time and country perhaps, the ladies were more temperate than they were in other ages and in other places. We find the gout a familiar disease among the Roman ladies; which Seneca, in his ninety fifth epistle justly ascribes to the luxurious living and debaucheries in which they indulged without control (p. 247).

The appearance of gout in Roman women may have resulted, like colic, from their increasing consumption of lead-laden wine. A fifth-century translation of Soranus of Ephesus (117–38 A.D.) makes it clear that the Greeks not only recognized gout but suspected wine to be a cause (24). The cure propounded by Soranus was severe. To the basic disapproval of self-indulgence he added a caution against licentiousness. "Have the patient strengthen his body by walking without shoes and by avoiding anything which might be harmful, that is to say, excesses of any kind, particularly of wine, indigestion and venery" (pp. 929–30). In the thirteenth century this venerable theory was repeated by Petrus Hispanus, who was to become Pope John XXI. "Muche surfettynge and dronke-nesse, to much accompaninge wyth women, imoderate exercise, long standynge, and such lyke," were the causes of gout recognized by this medieval pope-physician (404).

Medical opinion was couched in equivocation. In 1584, Thomas Cogan advised, "for one that hath the gowt, to forbeare wine and women," but then repeated the ancient lore, "Drinke wine and haue the gowt, drinke none and haue the gowt" (148, p. 4). Lazarus Riverius writing in 1653 listed among the causes of gout (643):

> All things which encrease raw and wheyish Humors, or any bad Humors whatsoever: as meats of gross substance hard to be digested, and such as afford many Excrements, frequent Gluttony and Drunkeness; immoderate Carnal Embracements which is the reason that Gout is called the Daughter of Bacchus and Venus (p. 533).

Condemning these perennial vices, Dr. Edward Baynard was moved to verse. In a letter to Sir John Floyer dated 1707, he mused, "Women and Wine, with Idleness alone, / Are the first Parents of the Gout and Stone" (262, p. 301).

While gout was not considered exactly a venereal disease, it was widely held to be one of the more debilitating consequences of copulation (659). Venereal disease was, on the other hand, in all its protean manifestations, seen as similar to gout. The French pox (syphilis) was called by some "the gout of the privicies." The connection between gout and Venus persists in the layman's mind. One journalist, writing recently of the "Agonies and Ecstasies of Gout," described the dependence of his libido on gout (709). Relief from the noxious assault on his great toe apparently undermined his potency. "I prefer an occasional twinge of gout—easily squelched by colchicine" (p. 81), Mr. Steinberg reports in *Esquire*, "to a life-time of diminished sex drive." To preserve the delights of Venus, this reporter avoids a cure.

Born of experience and the educated guess, pathophysiology remained an intuitive rather than an experimental art. As in modern times, the demands of practice rarely left time for rigorous verification of clinical judgment. Accuracy, a chancy business at best, seems all the more remarkable when viewed retrospectively. According to Copeman, the first English treatise on the gout dates from 1534 and was entitled *On Whether it is Possible to Cure the Gout or No* by Dominicus Burgauer. This early tract warns against "inordinate eating and drinking, mixing one's wines. . . . Also, drinking a lot of white wine on an empty stomach and using vinegar aids its [the gout's] acquisition" (158, p. 289). In addition to dietary discretion, secret concoctions and amulets are highly recommended.

In sixteenth-century England, Philip Barrough reiterated the ancient views, but in addition, linked colic with wine and the gout (43).

This disease is engendered of continual crudities and drunkeness and of immoderate using of lecherie. Also many times the cholicke being naughtely cured, is wont to be a cause why the joint sickness should follow. But for the most part, a disposition to this kinde of disease proceedeth from the parents to the children, and their posteritie. Let him abstaine altogether from flesh except in the birds of the mountaines. Let him use fishes that brede in stoney waters. Wine, if the intemperence of the sicke may suffer it, must altogether be taken away: for it is almost the only reason whereby health should follow: which seeing among a thousand, scarce one doth observe, it is not marvell though there be very fewe, which are delivered from this disease at these days (p. 212).

Barrough's discussion of gout includes colic and cites abstention from wine as the preferred mode of therapy. In addition to setting the stage for the English association of wine with gout, these two elements suggest that lead in wine was not uncommon in England centuries before it was recognized as a cause of colic or gout. Barrough's concern with the sources of protein in the diet similarly anticipated recognition of nutritive precursors (purines) of uric acid (363).

If the association of wine with colic, gout, and kidney stones sometimes appeared to be wholly fortuitous, therapy seemed little more than random health hints. A fifteenth-century translation of the *Secreta Secretorum*, purporting to be the sage advice given to a youthful Alexander the Great, asserts that he who gets plenty of sleep will be protected from abdominal pains and "shall nought drede goutys" (706, p. 77). The 1608 poem by John Harrington offers herbal cures. *The Englishman's Doctor or the Schoole of Salerne or Physicall Observations for the Perfect Preserving of the Body of Man in Continuall Health* brought ninth-century wisdom from the Medical School of Salerno to England. Largely a compilation of commonsense advice on diet, the verses also deal with the relationship between wine, colic, and the gout (356).

> Tho Nettles stinke, yet make they recompence,
> If you belly by the Collicke paine endures,
> Against the Collicke Nettle-seed and hony
> Is Physick: better none is had for money.
> It breedeth sleepe, staies vomits, fleams doth soften,
> It helpes him of the Gowte that eates it often.

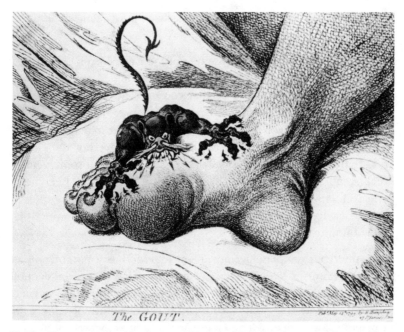

The GOUT.

15. The Gout, *engraved by James Gillray in 1799 demonstrates the conviction of personal experience. New York Public Library Prints Division.*

A bit later Harrington offers some final advice: "And some affirm that they haue found by tryall, / The paine of Gowt is cur'd by Penny-royall" (p. 119).

During the early Christian era, gout was viewed as retribution duly visited upon the sinful. Indeed, Gillray's well known image of *The Gout* suggests the Devil incarnate (fig. 15). Rodnan has identified no less than thirteen Christian saints, canonized prior to the thirteenth century, who counted among their miraculous powers the ability to cure the gout (650). The gouty were advised to direct their prayers to St. Genow and St. Maur while St. Erasmus was reputed to bring relief to the colic (601). When divine cures failed, resort was made to magic. Paracelsus prescribed amulets of fused lead, gold, silver, and iron to ward off the evil malady. The amulets were inscribed with signs of the "conjunction of Saturn and Mars" (lead and iron) for maximum astrological impact. The sixteenth-century alchemist did not suggest that the ingredients of his talisman could be numbered among the causes of the gout. He attributed gout to the "tartarous" residues of wine.

To the Puritan minister Cotton Mather, gout was a welcome penance, divine retribution (651). In 1724, he chastised gouty sinners as follows (516):

> Examine Syr, whether your Gout be not the natural probable effect of some intemperance, wherein you have indulged yourself; and consider your Ways. It may be that you have not been so careful about your Diet as you should have been. It may be you have the Tartar of the Wine you have drunk, sticking to your Joints; or it may be, as Hippocrates observed so long ago, Men have not the Gout before the Use of Venus, you may charge yourself with some venereal Irregularities. If you find any of this Guilt upon you, it becomes you to humble yourself before the Glorious God; humbly confess and bewayl your sinful Follies; humbly accept the Punishment of your Iniquity (p. 122).

The American temperance movement emerged as a potent political force two centuries later. The occasional presence of lead in alcoholic drinks increased the hazard of excessive drinking. The debilitating effects of alcohol on both individual health and social structure became a subject of enduring concern. The Americans, of course, were not alone in their ambivalence toward these beverages. Death also lurked in the Englishman's punch bowl (fig. 16).

None had more of the reformers' zeal than gouty old George Cheyne, who believed that all ailments stemmed from the evil brews (136).

> I would not hesitate a Moment, to ascribe to fermented and distill'd Liquors of any kind, the whole blame of all or most of the painful and excruciating Distempers that afflict Mankind: It is to it alone that all our Gouts, Stones, Cancers, Fevers, high Hysterics, Lunacy and Madness, are principally owing. It is the true Pandora's box (p. lvii).

Torn between venerating classical authority and scientific aspirations, Cheyne vacillated between paraphrasing ancient aphorisms and gathering anecdotes, but he never doubted that wine was responsible for the gout and its complications: colic, neurological symptoms, and kidney stones. His expertise in this area extended beyond theory to the taverns of London, where he had misspent much of his youth (414). Cheyne however, favored Boerhaave's view that the worst thing you could do for a gouty patient was relieve his pain. He recommended French claret which, in his experience, was likely to induce a paroxysm of gout, thereby avoiding "misplaced" gout (135). Forced by illness to retire to Bath from

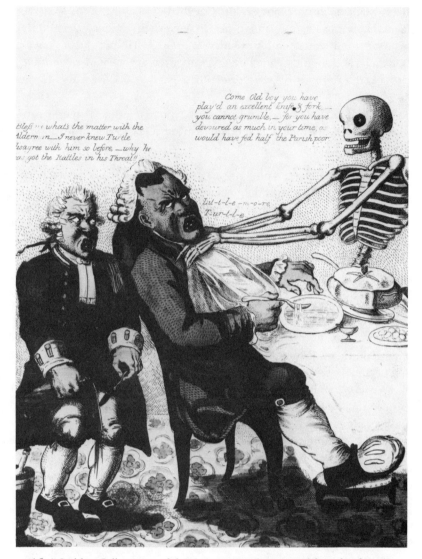

16. A Sudden Call, or one of the Corporation Summoned from his favorite Amusement, *anonymous engraving published by S. W. Fores, 1799. Death calls for the gouty glutton. From the collection of the National Library of Medicine.*

his Falstaffian existence in London, Cheyne became one of the spa's most fashionable physicians. Among his distinguished patients were Samuel Johnson, John Wesley, and Alexander Pope (414). His belief that gout was beneficial and should be encouraged rather than prevented, nevertheless provoked a dubious response; ridicule as well as reknown was his fate (494, 720).

The gout indeed proved a mighty disincentive to drink. Thomas Trotter was grateful that this affliction could provide at least some motivation for abstinence (753).

> As example is therefore better than precept, the juvenile debauchee should be occasionally introduced into the sick chamber of the hoary veteran in excess. If the children in Lacedaemon were to be trained to temperance, by looking on the disgusting actions and revelry of drunken slaves, let the youths of the present time be instructed from the unwieldy joints, withered limbs, and hypochondriacal glooms of our modern Arthritics (p. 115).

Under the presidency of John Collins Warren, the Massachusetts Temperance Society published a prize-winning essay by Dr. William B. Carpenter on the medical consequences of alcohol (119). Among the many additional accomplishments of John Collins Warren were the founding of the Massachusetts General Hospital and the *New England Journal of Medicine*, and the outlawing of the sale of intoxicating beverages in Boston on Sundays (337). Like Cheyne a century earlier, there were few human ailments that Carpenter did not attribute to drink. In addition to gout he considered kidney disease an inevitable consequence of excessive "stimulation" from alcohol. Carpenter anticipated later biochemical studies by hypothesizing a mediating role for lactic acid in the induction of gout.

Although wine and gout have long been associated, the causal relationship remains controversial. Gout has not been produced in experimental animals and, indeed, occurs spontaneously in man even in the absence of hyperuricemia or lead poisoning. Too many variables are involved to permit designation of a single cause. A confluence of correlations, nevertheless, implies causation when no single link is compelling. Epidemics of gout appearing sporadically throughout the ages have been related to fermented drinks. The association with palsies, colic, and encephalopathy suggests the role of lead even though the etiology was not recognized in the original description.

From the earliest times, descriptions of gout were picturesque. One sixteenth-century scholar wrote (814), "The name Podagra is naught els, but a snare wherewith birds be catched by their feete, and therefore is this disease of the gout likened to that instrument; for that it doth catch men by the feete, and holdeth them caught therewith" (p. 540). Early accounts were rarely precisely limited to a specific form of arthritis. Nevertheless, they often had the distinguishing conviction of personal experience. Gout's signature was the exquisite pain in the great toe. In A.D. 135 Aretaeus wrote (157), "No other pain is more severe than this, not iron screws, nor cords, not the wound of a dagger, nor burning fire" (p. 34).

In the sixteenth century, Ambrose Paré emphasized the extreme suffering: "through the vehemency of the agony many are almost mad and wish themselves dead" (157, p. 53). But Sydenham was the most eloquent in his classic description of 1683 (724).

> About midnight the agony is at its worst. Now it is a violent stretching and tearing of the ligaments—now it is a gnawing pain, like that of a dog, and now a pressure and tightening. So exquisite and lively meanwhile is the feeling of the part affected, that the sufferer cannot bear the weight of the bed-clothes nor the jar of a person walking into the room. The pain is not abated before two or three o'clock in the morning the next day (p. 300).

In addition to the memorable prose, the singular directness of Sydenham's description distinguished his perception of nature from that of his predecessors. His omission of the metaphysical was as important as the precision of his observation. But it was the fluidity of his language which made Sydenham the leader of the renaissance in English medicine. While not an experimentalist, Sydenham shared the glory of the founders of English science—William Harvey, Isaac Newton, and Robert Boyle. His views on etiology were, however, conventional. "The gout generally attacks those aged persons, who have spent most part of their lives in ease, voluptuousness, high living and too free an use of wine, and other spiritous liquors" (724, p. 181).

According to Sydenham: "Those symptoms which threaten the life of a patient must be met. Of such the commonest is languor of the stomach with gripes, as if from Wind" (724, p. 304). For his own part, Sydenham had "recourse to laudanum" (p. 249), small beer, and Iberian wine. Despite his choice of therapy, Sydenham thought wine dangerous to gouty patients. Of therapy he wrote, "Riding on horseback is best" (p. 303). But also the ancient prohibition, "Gouty men must not indulge in venery" (p. 303).

In England, treatises on the gout flowered with the same fecundity as tophi. All of Britain, it seems, was stricken. "And I doubt very much," observed Sir William Temple in 1680, "whether the great encrease of that Disease in England within these twenty years, may so have been occasioned by the custom of much Wine introduced in our Constant and Common Tables" (737, p. 236). English martyrdom to the gout became increasingly debilitating in the eighteenth century (648). "The Gout of late Years has mightily encreased amongst us here in England; and that we have had more gouty People, within the Compass of ten Years past, than ever were known before, in so short a Period of Time" (p. lv). "'Tis amazing to think, what Havoc the Gout makes in the present Century, in this part of the World;" wrote R. Drake of London, "so much that it has become kind of a popular Disease; and I think the Expression just, in calling it an English Plague" (A2, p. vi).

William Cadogen's preaching received particular notoriety. Despite his stated allegiance to the scientific method, Cadogen's concept of the gout was wholly theoretical. He recognized three causes (110).

> Indolence, Intemperence and Vexation . . . [p. 19].
>
> In England all degrees of men are furnished with the means of intemperance, and therefore it is no wonder that most men are intemperate.
>
> . . . I verily believe that there are more gouts in England, than in all the rest of Europe: a proof that good living is more universal [p. 39].
>
> . . . It will be said, that many drink wine every day without gout, stone or any disease at all in consequence of it. I believe not many, or I should know some of them [p. 48].

In lieu of a cure and as compensation for the suffering of the intemperate, patients were assured that gout was an affliction of the privileged classes. In "the Physician's Consolation on the Gout," Daniel Sennert offered a fabulous tale showing how the Gout came to be "the Rich-Man's Disease" (679). Rambling about the countryside, the fable goes, Gout found "nothing but little cottages, most rudely and unhandsomely built and very fithily scituated; and could find there nothing but Mattocks and Pitchforks, Rakes and suchlike rustical instruments." Rejecting these vulgar surroundings, Gout then rambled about the city. Here she found "nothing but Jollity and Feasting . . . the house of Ease and Idleness" and, Gout concluded, "This is indeed the House and this the Palace that is fit for my Reception and Entertainment" (p. 7).

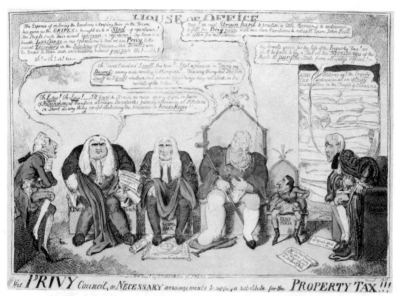

17. The Privy Council, or Necessary arrangements to supply a substitute for
the Property Tax !!! *The gouty prince regent, later George IV, shares
the gripes with his councilors. Engraving by George Cruikshank, 1816.
Copyright British Museum.*

Wine and gout incapacitated England's finest. The belief that gout
occurs mainly in the wealthy and powerful was loudly proclaimed by
Sydenham (723).

> But what is a consolation to me, and may be so to other gouty
> persons of small fortunes and slender abilities, is, that kings,
> princes, generals, admirals, philosophers, and several other great
> men, have thus lived and died. In short, it may in a more especial
> manner be affirmed of this disease, that it destroys more rich than
> poor persons, and more wise men than fools; . . . so that it appears
> to be universally and absolutely decreed that no man shall enjoy
> unmixed happiness or misery, but experience both (pp. 193–94).

Crippling arthritis of the foot was not the only disease which hounded
the upper classes. The failure of bodily functions symbolized the popular
perception of the failure of government. For George IV, podagra and
kidney stones were compounded by humiliating stomach pains (figs.
17–18). That lead may have been responsible for the king's torment is
suggested by the memoirs of the duke of Buckingham, in which it is re-

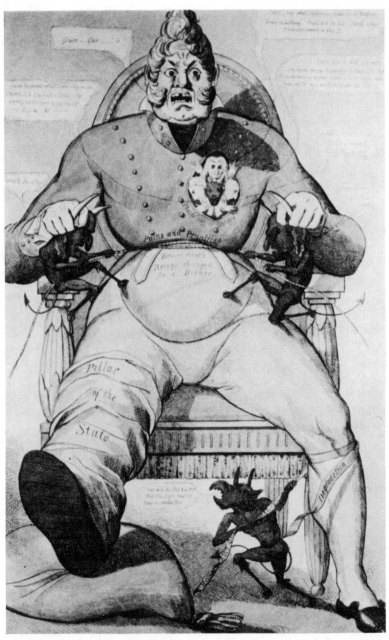

18. The Brightest Star in the State . . . or . . . A Peep out of the Royal Window. *The ailments of George IV include gout and "Pains and Penalties" of the stomach. Engraving by George Cruikshank, 1820. From the collection of William Helfand.*

corded, that George IV, as prince regent, suffered temporary palsies in his arms in 1811 (109).

The protean illnesses of the royal family have led to interesting modern speculations on etiology. In addition to suffering from gout and abdominal colic, George III was generally believed to be insane. Impressive arguments have been mustered suggesting that the father of George IV suffered from a rare genetic disorder, hepatic porphyria (481, 482). The evidence has been interpreted as indicating that the ancestors and descendants of George III transmitted this metabolic defect over four centuries. It has, however, become increasingly clear that a number of environmental toxins can induce similar clinical and biochemical abnormalities. Lead and alcohol are the best known of the chemical agents which contribute to the clinical expression of porphyria. It is perhaps not just coincidence that both porhyria and plumbism occur among the alcoholics consigned to psychiatric wards (411).

A. B. Garrod's son had a hand in devising a practical method for detecting lead poisoning. Using a crude spectrophotometric method in 1892, A. E. Garrod reported the presence of "hematoporphyrin" in the urine of a patient with gout (293). This compound was later called uro- or coproporphyrin (782). The younger Garrod believed that urinary excretion of hematoporphyrin was the result of associated liver disease (294), but, in retrospect, saturnine gout seems as likely a diagnosis. Today the younger Garrod's fame rests on coining the phrase "inborn error of metabolism" to describe gout. He was less attuned to secondary causes of gout.

Urinary hematoporphyrin excretion in lead intoxication was first reported in 1895 (716). By the middle of the present century, heme precursors in urine and blood had become the most important biochemical indicators of both lead poisoning and hepatic porphyria (198). Porphyria is a rather esoteric metabolic disease involving aberrant hemoglobin synthesis and at times resulting in unnecessary abdominal surgery.

The similarities between lead poisoning and porphyria assure some diagnostic confusion. Lead poisoning mimics porphyria in its major clinical manifestations—colic, palsy, and encephalopathy (176, 279). Symptomatic plumbism is distinguished from porphyria by the presence of anemia and specific heme pigments in the urine. In plumbism the major pigment is coproporphyrin, while in hepatic porphyria, the major urinary pigment is porphobilinogen. Urinary porphobilinogen has a striking propensity to turn the color of port wine when exposed to sunlight. The red-purple hue results from the oxidation of porphobilinogen to porphyrin in the presence of oxygen and sunlight in an acidic solution. Such burgundy-blue urine could not go unnoticed even in the eighteenth century. The occasional recording of bizarrely colored urine voided by George III was the key to the retrospective diagnosis of familial porphyria (481).

There is, however, overlap in urinary excretion patterns of plumbism and porphyria (280), and port wine–colored urine has occasionally been noted in lead intoxication (167, 310, 343, 716, 782). In recent decades an increasing number of similarities between environmentally and genetically acquired diseases have been noted. Hypertension and renal disease, long associated with plumbism, have been reported to be common among porphyrics in South Africa (184, 197, 211). Conversely, the dramatic blistering of the skin characteristic of porphyria cutanea tarda in South Africa has been observed among lead-poisoned patients in Britain (16, A3) and among renal dialysis patients in South Africa (183). Excessive drinking is accepted as the most common inciting cause in South African patients with porphryia (197). Because of the skin lesions noted in some members of the royal family, Macalpine and Hunter seem to have modified their diagnosis from acute intermittent porphyria to variegate porphyria, a choice which takes into account the dermatologic signs in the royal progeny (482).

The similarities between lead poisoning and the porphyrias raise the possibility that the diagnosis may depend more on the conceptual heritage of physicians than the genetic heritage of patients. As long as the diagnosis of lead poisoning is based on the patients' knowledge of exposure and blood lead levels, lead poisoning is likely to be overlooked even by the most experienced of physicians. Urinary porphobilinogen is sometimes increased in symptomatic lead poisoning (184, 197, 431, 606). But other heme precursors can also produce startling colors in the urine and the chemical nature of these colorful compounds is not always known (Manfred Doss, personal communication).

Thomas Oliver found that the urine in lead poisoning turned bright red or blue when treated with acid (563). He called the color-producing compound "indican," and found it was soluble in chloroform. The ability of urobilinogen to spontaneously turn urine dark red stimulated Watson and Schwartz to develop their famous test for porphobilinogen by virtue of its solubility in chloroform and red fluorescence in ultraviolet light (782).

Not only are the manifestations of plumbism and porphyria almost indistinguishable, but the methods of treatment are often identical. The chelating agent EDTA has been reported to be remarkably effective in both conditions (197). The mechanism of its efficacy in plumbism is well

known; EDTA removes lead from the body. In porphyria it has been theo-
rized that the therapeutic effect is due to the removal of zinc or copper.
These metals are indeed excreted in very large quantities during chelation treatment, so much so that in porphyria the effect of chelation on
lead has received only cursory attention (195). Theoretical considerations about zinc and copper are reported in detail while lead is alluded to
only in footnotes (600). Renal disease has recently been designated a
new precipitating cause of porphyria although no attempt was made to
rule out unrecognized lead poisoning (185). Systematic studies of body
lead stores in patients with porphyria have yet to be performed. Elabo-
rate theories of genetic transmission of metabolic defects would appear
to hold more fascination for modern researchers than do mundane measurements. The response of porphyria patients to chelation therapy suggests that some of these sufferers, too, may harbor lead poisoning in
disguise.

Misdiagnosis of lead poisoning as porphyria is by no means unknown
even in the most sophisticated of contemporary medical circles (68, 198,
593). The congenital porphyria in Britain's royal family might, therefore,
warrant a second look. The secret of the king's madness, like Newton's,
may yet reside within his bones.

Macalpine discounted lead poisoning as the cause of the royal affliction
with the following footnote (481):

> Lead poisoning, which also causes colic, palsy, and encephalopa-
> thy, can be excluded by absence of anaemia and presence of tachy-
> cardia; and distinct attacks over many years without other members
> of the household being affected. Nor would Sir George Baker have
> missed plumbism, since it was he who demonstrated that lead poi-
> soning was the cause of "the endemial colic of Devonshire" (p. 69).

Could Sir George Baker have overlooked lead toxicity in King George
III? The answer is most certainly yes—particularly the delayed sequelae
of prolonged exposure. It should be remembered that Baker had not recorded cerebral symptoms among the signs of the Devonshire colic.
Baker omitted encephalopathy from his description of lead poisoning
just as he omitted saturnine gout and nephropathy. Anemia was not, of
course, determined quantitatively in those days, and pallor might well
have seemed unremarkable in so gravely ill and grand a personnage.
Tachycardia, on the other hand, is hardly sufficiently specific to establish
the diagnosis of porphyria. King James I, George III's forebear, suffered
similar symptoms, associated in James' case with kidney stones, con-

firmed post-mortem (482). Kidney stones are of course, more characteristic of gout than of hereditary porphyria.

The crucial "blue" urine passed by George III could have been due to
lead rather than the rarer and more esoteric "inborn error of metabolism." Insidious lead poisoning can reasonably explain gout, as well as
strangely colored urine; hereditary porphyria cannot. It has been said,
"When you hear hoofbeats, don't look for zebras" (Marvin F. Levitt, M.D.,
personal communication). Colic, palsy, and the gout are the hoofbeats
of lead.

Such hindsight may seem idle speculation, but the question is not beyond resolution. The exclusion of lead as the cause of the royal malady
requires only the measurement of lead content in the royal bones. A positive finding might remove from historical footnotes the hereditary taint
of royal consanguinity and substitute a regal appetite for port. England's
stillbirths and sterility, gout and colic might have had the same cause as
Rome's. While lead now seems suspect, wine was for centuries deemed
the universal culprit, views which are by no means mutually exclusive.
Insidious lead poisoning may well have caused colic, insanity, kidney
stones, and gout in the British royal family.

Alfred Baring Garrod concurred in the traditional view that drinking
caused the gout (289). "There is no truth in medicine better established
than the fact that the use of fermented or alcoholic liquors is the most
powerful of all the predisposing causes of gout; nay so potent, that it may
be a question whether gout would ever have been known to mankind
had such beverages not been indulged in" (p. 260). Wine consumption
also precipitated attacks of gouty arthritis, probably related to transient
elevations of serum uric acid. Thus, wine was associated with acute paroxysms as well as chronic gout. So dramatic were the immediate effects that
Garrod used a gout attack in response to alcohol as a confirmatory, diagnostic test (289). This provocative test for gout has not entirely gone out
of fashion (432). Its effectiveness may be explained by acute elevations
of serum uric acid levels resulting from alcohol and fasting, which transiently diminish the renal excretion of uric acid (492).

The idea that gout victimizes the privileged and intellectual classes in
particular persists to this day (209). Next to drinking and venery, scholarship was most suspect as a predisposing cause (99). All the accouter-
ments of the scholarly dilettante are present in an 1827 caricature of the
consequences of "enlarged understanding": wine, books, art, crutches,
and a gout stool (fig. 19). A middle-age paunch and the gout adorn this
middling student. One modern professor of medicine reports he has

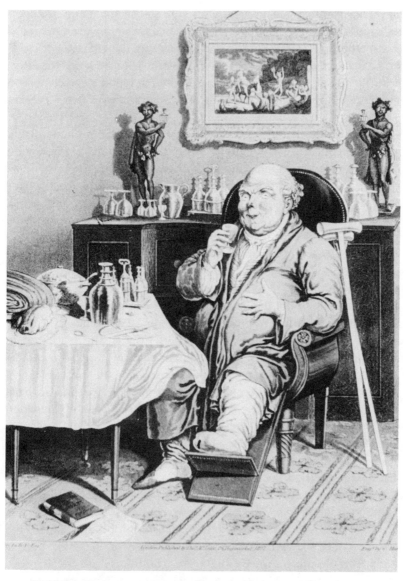

19. The typical gout patient had An Exquisite Taste, with an Enlarged Understanding *which included the finest Portuguese wines. Drawn by "E.Y.," engraved by George Hunt, 1827. From the author's collection.*

"never seen gout in persons with a low I.Q." Similar, if not quite compelling, support for such vanity derives from research employing more fastidious methods (321). Analyzing data from many individuals, Fessel observed that college students have higher serum uric acid levels than their nonacademic peers (257), while DeWitt Stetten found a correlation between intelligence and serum uric acid levels among Army recruits (710).

While the idea that the diverse life-styles of scholars and gourmands both cause gout strains credulity, recent physiologic studies lend support to these associations. A multiplicity of factors determines who, when, and where acute gouty arthritis will strike. Experimental evidence of the effect of posture on uric acid confirms the most ancient concepts of gout. The term itself means "drop," in French, originating from the Latin "gutta"—to run down. According to humoral theory, Phlegme, arising in the pituitary body, is dispersed to the great toe, thereby inciting acute gouty attacks (644). The morbific matter would indeed appear to drop into the great toe under appropriate conditions.

The susceptibility of the great toe seems to be related to the dependent position of the feet when sitting or standing. Fluid tends to accumulate in this joint under the pressure of gravity. Inactivity further increases this accumulation. Upon reclining, the joint fluid returns to the circulation followed, more slowly, by uric acid. Consequently, in the early morning hours, the concentration of uric acid temporarily rises in synovial fluid. The relatively low temperature of the extremity in combination with the elevated local uric acid level nurtures urate crystal precipitation. However, this is only one of many incompletely understood biophysical factors which regulate crystal formation in joint fluid. The base of the great toe is particularly vulnerable to these events because of the constant trauma it sustains over years of normal walking.

A sudden fall in joint-fluid uric acid concentration may also result in release of uric acid crystals. Here the mechanism does not require the formation of new crystals but, rather, their release into the joint space as uric acid tophi are resorbed (485, 688). The release of crystals previously fixed to tissue is believed to be the cause of the acute attacks of gout commonly occurring during allopurinol therapy.

Swings in serum uric acid concentration are exacerbated by irregularities of diet. Food rich in uric acid precursors may transiently increase uric acid formation and decrease renal excretion, raising serum levels after large meals (492). When combined with alcohol, such sudden fluctuations predispose to crystal formation and release, and hence to gouty attacks. One can readily imagine how the sedentary life of the scholar creates an ideal setting for these physiologic events.

By the end of the eighteenth century Wollaston had identified lithic acid in tophi. In 1797 Pearson proposed that the term "lithic," derived by Scheele (650) from "lithiasis" in 1776, be replaced by "uric" and the later appellation held (587). The presence of uric acid crystals in the urine of gouty patients had been described by Scheele in 1786. Despite these advances, the nature of gout remained problematic. Sir Charles Scudamore, the foremost English authority on gout prior to Garrod, subscribed to traditional concepts. He doubted the growing body of evidence pointing to uric acid as the metabolic signature of gout. He did not believe that uric acid was important because patients with tophi were relatively rare and, furthermore, uric acid was found in abundance in the urine of nongouty patients.

According to Garrod, who attended Sir Charles during his terminal illness, Scudamore relinquished traditional doctrine for the evidence of chemistry only toward the end of his life (290). Nevertheless, in his salad days, Scudamore further confused the issues by deploring what he believed to be exaggerated claims for colchicine (677). Although severe abdominal pains were frequent in his patients, Scudamore did not consider lead a possible cause of their complaints.

Scudamore favored the traditional therapies for gout including mercury, venesection, cupping, poultices, sarsaparilla, and ass's milk. If these remedies met with the patient's displeasure, he advocated a visit to Britain's favorite spa. The solace of Bath had the sanction of long pharmacologic tradition for the treatment of gout as well as colic. "I am fully persuaded," declared Nicolas Robinson in 1755, "that no other Fluid so readily dissolves the gouty Salts, and discharges them by Perspiration, as the Bath-Waters" (648, p. 139). Few recommendations for the treatment of gout have received more popular acceptance by the affluent. The spectacle of Bath as a watering place for the gouty bourgeoisie was a familiar subject of caricature by Thomas Rowlandson. The swollen foot swathed in flannel, delicately perched on a gout stool, was the nineteenth-century cartoonist's metaphor for overindulgence. The coddled foot became a familiar symbol in the works of Cruikshank, Gillray, and Heath. Sustained across oceans and time, Uncle Sam's political maladies were also symbolized by the bandaged foot (fig. 20). The pictorial language persists in a 1979 *Archie* comic portraying the moral decay of the affluent upper classes (fig. 21).

While the Bath waters were undoubtedly more restorative to the spirit

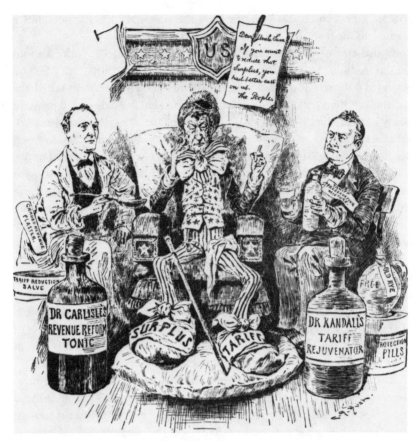

20. *The gouty foot, hallmark of British caricature, was sometimes used in American political satire.* Uncle Sam and His Doctors *appeared as an engraving by C. G. Bush in* Harper's Weekly, *October 22, 1887. From the author's collection.*

than to the metabolism, the introduction of biological chemistry into the practice of medicine provided an understanding of how the mineral waters might prevent the complications of gout. Henry Bence-Jones pointed out that alkali introduced into the body by such waters would increase the solubility of uric acid in urine and hence decrease stone formation and improve excretion (60). While this hypothesis seems valid, it is unlikely that significant alkalinization of the urine can be achieved unless enormous quantities of alkaline mineral waters are consumed.

Regional as well as class differences in the incidence of gout made it

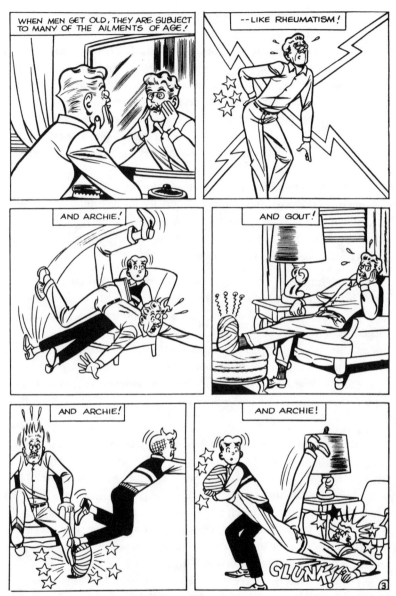

21. Contemporary comics still use the gouty foot to symbolize upper-class decadence. From Archie Annual Digest No. 35 *(1979),* © *1983, Archie Comic Publications, Inc.*

impossible for English physicians to agree on the role of alcohol. Drinking was ubiquitous but the gout seemed to favor certain geographic areas. Attempts were made to explain the variable prevalence of gout by the type of alcoholic beverage consumed. Epidemiologic studies conducted largely by hearsay led to the conclusion that certain alcoholic drinks actually were beneficial to the gout. Scudamore noted that, "in Glasgow the gout is very rare, even amongst the higher classes. . . . In Glasgow, also, punch is a more general beverage at the best tables than wine. Hence I often heard it facetiously remarked, 'that punch keeps off the gout'" (676, p. 42).

Increasing resistance to abstinence combined with strong personal preference on the part of some physicians led to flexibility in the gout regimen. Opinions might even have been influenced by competition for wealthy patients. Not to be misunderstood as favoring abstinence, Wainewright extoled the virtues of drink (772).

> Though Excess in strong Liquors be so prejudicial, yet the moderate Use of them are often of great Advantage; and certainly they are great Blessings to Mankind. . . . How comforting is a Glass of some grateful spiritous Liquor? It blunts the Sense of Pain, exhilarates the dropping Spirits, banishes Melancholy satisfies hunger, when Victuals are not to be had; 'tis useful in all Distempers where the Pulse is low, where the Blood abounds with Serum, where Perspiration is surpressed, and where the Passions of Mind are Violent (pp. 221–22).

Despite recognition of the association of wine with gout, liquor was often recommended in the treatment of the very symptoms of gout, which, in retrospect, were probably due to adulterants. William Cullen was quite specific in his recommendations for gout of the stomach (172). "When this affects the stomach and intestines, relief is to be instantly attempted by the free use of strong wines, joined with aromatics, and given warm; or if these shall not prove enough, ardent spirits must be employed, and are to be given in a large dose" (p. 283).

The popular tendency to reverse causality moved Ben Jonson to write "Bacchus Turn'd Doctor," a verse of which claims (747):

> Some have Tisick, some have Rheume,
> Some have Palsy, some have Gout,
> Some swell with Fat, and some sonsume,
> But they are sound that drink all out.

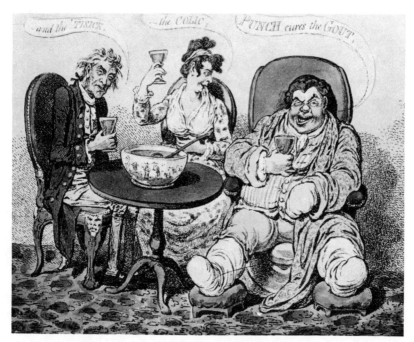

22. Punch Cures the Gout, *companion piece to James Gillray's* The Gout
*(fig. 15) of 1799. The saturnine components of this dismal feast include rum
punch (lead-laden?), the colic, and cachexia. From the collection of the
New York Public Library.*

'Tis Wine, Pure Wine, Revives sad Souls
Therefore give us Chearing Bowls.

Drawn at the same time as *The Gout* (fig. 15), Gillray's *Punch Cures the
Gout* shows the full range of the pathophysiologic concomitants of this
ubiquitous condition (fig. 22). The characters recite the doggerel they
illustrate; "Punch cures the Gout, the Colic, and the 'Tisick," appears in
the balloons. The verse continues, though not shown: "And is by all
agreed the very best of physic" (820, p. 449).

In addition to showing the venerable association wtih drinking, we see
that colic closely followed the gout. At that time colic was viewed as "irregular" or "retrocedent" gout; the morbid process was believed to have
left the great toe to strike the internal organs. Today such extra-articular
symptoms are better interpreted as lead poisoning. The association of
gout, colic, and wine was probably due to the presence of lead in the
punch. While "'tisic" referred primarily to consumption (phthisis), ema-

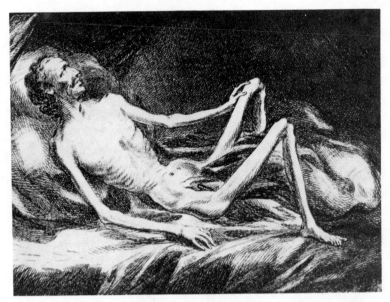

23. *Lead cachexia, illustrated in Ebell's work, published in 1794, on lead poisoning among glaziers in eighteenth-century Germany (212).*

ciation of any cause often was so termed. In this setting it seems likely that lead-laden punch had caused wasting as well as colic and gout. The grim figure of lead cachexia, described so vividly by Citois, had been illustrated in 1794 by Ebell (fig. 23, [212]) and was familiar in Europe. In short, Gillray's cartoon depicts major consequences of alcoholic beverages adulterated with lead and satirizes the reversal of cause and effect evident in popular practice.

Gillray's fantasy struck a responsive chord; it was republished frequently. Although the rhyme and figures varied, the message remained the same (fig. 24). "Punch is good for gout; for more gout more punch is good" went one aphorism (788). At times, wine took the spotlight: In *Champaign Driving Away Real Pain*, the afflicted recite, "Wine Cures the Gout, the Colic and the Phthsic/ Wine it is to all men the very Best of Physic" (fig. 25). Here, a servant gleefully pours gout medicines into the fire as counterpoint to the forced gaiety of the scene. When the physician ordered "Punch" for the treatment of gouty England, John Bull groaned, "Oh! Doctor! Doctor! *your Remedies* are worse than the Disease" (fig. 26).

Common wisdom mistook the cause for the cure. A bit of small warm punch was irresistible. Rum was recommended as the vehicle for gum

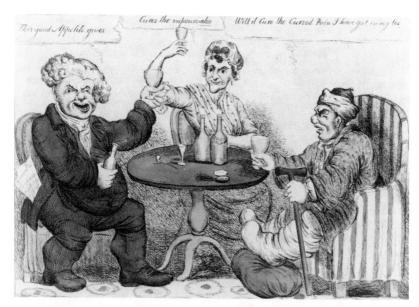

24. Palatable Physic, *engraved by William Heath in 1810, parodies Gillray's caricature (fig. 22). The gouty boozer asks, "Will it Cure the Cursed Pain I have got in my toe?" From the collection of the National Library of Medicine.*

guiacum therapy of podagra by one physician who assured his readers that the beverage could, in any case, not be worse for them than Portuguese wines (400). Another eighteenth-century physician, Thomas Short, considered rum particularly beneficial to the kidneys. His description of the renal effects of rum illustrates the contradictory and fanciful advice that evolved from anecdotal medicine; it exemplifies physiology founded on theory unfettered by observation (684). Dr. Short also recommended strong punch made with brandy or rum for the treatment of gout as "an Antidote against bilious Cholicks" (p. 192) and "gripes" (p. 195). "Paradoxical as it may appear," noted James Parkinson, "there is no doubt but that the practice of giving wine, with the intention of curing gout, has been sometimes adopted, in consequence of its having been sometimes successfully employed in producing this disease" (587, p. 123).

To the provincial American physician, brandy attained a reputation as an outstanding cure for the gout. In *The Planter's and Mariner's Medical Companion*, dedicated to Thomas Jefferson, James Ewell extolled the virtues of brandy with a burst of postrevolutionary fervor (248).

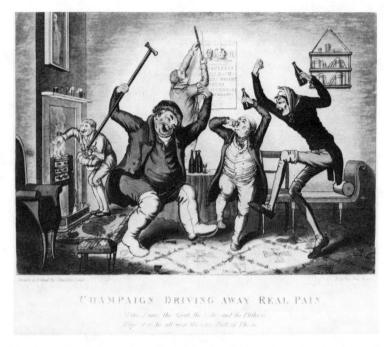

25. Champaign Driving Away Real Pain. *Another version of Gillray's* Punch Cures the Gout *(fig. 22) drawn by Theodore Lane and engraved by George Hunt, about 1827, in London. From the author's collection.*

For lack of this ammunition, the gallant Wayne was cut off long before "his eye was dim, or his natural heat abated." Late in the December of 1796, he embarked at Detroit for Presque Isle, but not without the usual supply of brandy, which, however, was all lost, through his servant's carelessness in upsetting his case. On the passage he caught cold which brought on a violent gout of the stomach; and, for want of his usual remedy, he suffered the most excruciating torture until he reached Presque Isle, where he died early in January, 1797. His body was deposited in the center of the fort, to show the children of future days, the grave of him, who so bravely defended their liberties (p. 149).

It is not surprising, then, to find that the perplexed patient soon came to view Madeira as the best cure for whatever ailed him (fig. 27). In the face of conflicting medical opinion, laymen followed their natural inclinations.

In a pamphlet on *The Use of Brandy and Salt as a Remedy* published in Boston in 1851, William lee offered his discovery for the cure of colic

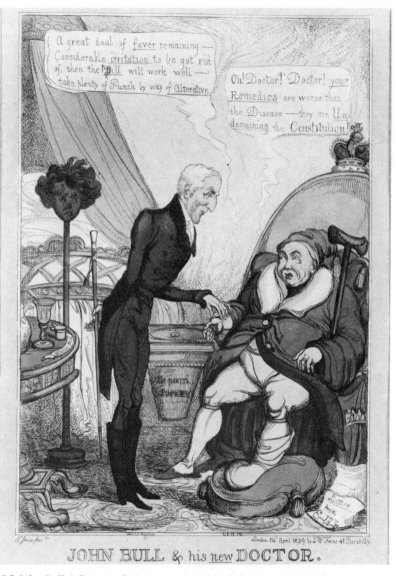

26. John Bull & his new Doctor, *engraved by J. Jones in 1829 indicts punch as the cause of George IV's malaise and (Dr.) Wellington's cure as worse than the disease. Copyright British Museum.*

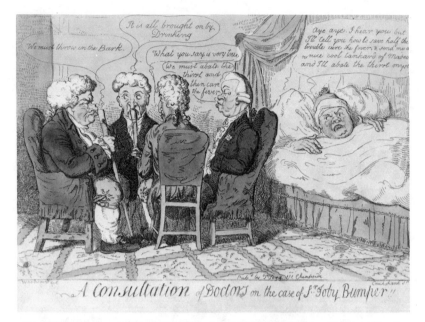

27. A Consultation of Doctors on the Case of Sir Toby Bumper!! *engraving by Isaac Cruikshank in 1807 suggests the reversal of causality in the popular mind. Despite the opinion of the learned doctors, the patient believes his only hope lies with Madeira. From the author's collection.*

and seventy-eight other ailments. For the gout he instructed, "the person afflicted should have his or her crown of the head well rubbed with the remedy" (450, p. 9).

Another pamphlet entitled *Wine in the Different Forms of Anemia and Atonic Gout* advocated wine as specific therapy for most conditions (55). The belief that alcoholic drink might be the cure rather than the cause of gout was a curious reversal of thinking which persisted into the twentieth century. An advertisement in *Harper's Weekly* of 1912 suggested that champagne may be particularly beneficial to the gout (fig. 28).

Sydenham rejected traditional purgative therapy although such medicine sometimes contained colchicine, the relatively specific antigout agent commonly used today. Despite his major contributions to the sound description of disease, Sydenham has been accused of removing this highly effective agent from medical practice. His enormous authority and personal conviction in this matter led to a loss of popularity of colchicine for almost two centuries (157).

The blame placed on Sydenham seems somewhat excessive when it is remembered that colchicine was only one of a vast potpourri of plants

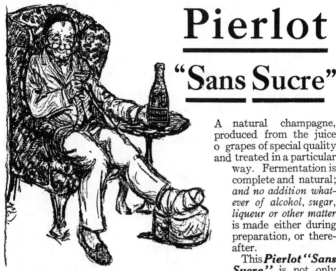
28. This advertisement for Pierlot of 1912 recommends this champagne for the treatment of gout. From the author's collection.

and herbs used since antiquity in magical potions. Hermodactyl and hellebore were reintroduced by Alexander of Tralles around A.D. 550 and again by Paracelsus in the sixteenth century. These plants are believed to be early names for the autumn crocus, whose roots contained colchicine as their active constituent (157, 291). The Elizabethan physician Philip Barrough recommended hermodactyl pills for purging gout patients. "Pilulae ex Hermodactylis," he wrote, "do retaine the ancient composition, and be of themselves . . . effectuall against the inveterate diseases of the joynts" (43, p. 444). By the seventeenth century any idea of a specific effect on gout had, however, been obscured by the more obnoxious cathartic side effects.

Prior to Sydenham, hermodactyl was regularly included among the salad of remedies recommended for arthritis. The unauthorized translation of the first English pharmacopoeia, the *Pharmacopoeia Londinensis: Or the London Dispensory*, "Pilule de Hermodactilis" (p. 141) contained sagapen, opopanax, coleworts, aloes, citron, myrobalans, turbith, coloquintida, bdellium, euphorbium, rue, smallage, castorium, sarcocol, saffrow, and honey as well as hermodactyls (173). The translator, Nicholas Culpeper, explained, "of Hermodactyls. They are hot and dry, purge phlegm, especially from the joynts, therefore are good for Gouts" (p. 7). Lazarus Riverius included the crocus in his potpourri of fifty-eight concoctions appearing before "Live Puppies applyed" but after "Sheeps dung" (644, p. 378). The chance inclusion of an effective agent was outweighed by a plethora of totally useless remedies. Sydenham's distrust of purgatives, based on bitter personal experience, consigned random, rather than rational, use of colchicine to obscurity.

Frustrated in all their attempts to cure the gout, creative physicians devised a meticulously reasoned strategy of therapeutic nihilism consistent with popular prejudice: the cure of gout was deemed detrimental to health and was the cause of irregular gout. Relief of the acute arthritis was generally conceded to be more dangerous than the disease itself. Since physicians, as an article of faith and self-esteem, could not believe the fault to be theirs, they agreed that the gout, displaced from the joints, would aggressively attack the other body organs. The wise physician avoided such dangerous displacements remembering Boerhaave's precept: "If the signs be present of the Gout being turned inwards, you must without delay attempt to drive it back into the joints."

Boerhaave's logic provided grounds for a conservative approach. Recommended in 1763 by Baron von Störck as a cure for dropsy (718), colchicum autumnale, the meadow saffron, found powerful opponents in the medical profession. Sold as a secret remedy by a somewhat shady French army officer, Husson, the English were not about to jump on the bandwagon of yet another panacea for gout, particularly a Frenchman's. Their skepticism was reinforced by the extravagant price demanded by Husson and the vast array of diseases (including lead poisoning) which he claimed this "universal specific" would cure (777). Edwin Jones created a sensation in London by reporting that Husson's Eau Medicinale, while not a universal cure, was indeed a specific for gout (409). Jones knew only that the secret formula was vegetable in origin and that patients who used it for catharsis found their gout mysteriously relieved within forty-eight hours. The Eau Medicinale was unfailing in curing the regular gout.

King George IV was soon extolling its virtues and the surgeon James Moore set about to determine the ingredients of the secret remedy. But, chemical analysis was not yet up to the task of discriminating between the myriad of organic materials that Husson incorporated into his concoction. Using little more than his sense of smell and uncanny intuition, Moore surmised that Eau Medicinale was a mixture of Sydenham's Vinous Laudanum (opium, saffron, cinnamon, and cloves in Spanish wine) and tincture of white hellebore (532). The most telling clue was, according to Moore, Husson's exorbitant claims plagiarized directly from Pliny; Husson asserted that the Eau Medicinale would cure madness but was ineffective in pulmonary diseases. Gout was but an afterthought—exactly as recorded by Pliny.

Undeterred by the effectiveness of Husson's secret remedy, the English took a firm stand against the use of the specific antigout drug (677). Effective treatment was deemed detrimental to health. The benefits of gout were clarified by Robertson (647).

> Interference with such paroxysms involves the increase of the greater evil,—risking not only the conversion of acute to irregular, or chronic gout, but the consequent deposition of chalky matter in the joints. . . . colchicum becomes an unjustifiable means of treatment, one that indirectly produces a greater evil than it relieves (pp. 245–46).

Even more subtle arguments against the use of colchicine were proffered by John Parkin who concluded that the drug was ineffective in the gout because it failed to relieve the symptoms of retrocedent gout (586).

Trapped by medical semantics, Parkin could not discern that the colchicine effect defined gout more accurately than the entire mass of treatises produced by self-proclaimed "gout doctors."

Before the specificity of Husson's Eau Medicinale became generally known, some practitioners thought they had identified its mechanism of action—purgation. On this basis, Thomas Sutton recommended calomel as an even better cathartic and reported that it was just as beneficial as Husson's higher-priced remedy for the alleviation of gout (721). "Any man, who relaxes in his endeavours to avert this disorder, in consequence of Husson's boasted discovery," wrote John Ring in 1811, ". . . ought indeed to be purged with Hellebore" (641, p. 207). Citing 5,623 deaths from gout in England between 1848 and 1868, Peter Hood contended that all of these fatalities were the result of too free use of colchicum (384).

The remarkable effectiveness of colchicine in gout remains the subject of modern investigation. In contrast to other anti-inflammatory agents such as aspirin and cortisone, the action of colchicine appears to be mediated by inhibition of a "crystal induced chemotactic factor" released by neutrophiles upon physical contact with urate crystals (701). Colchicine prevents the engulfing of crystals by white blood cells and the consequent pain and inflammation. Such details are, however, the preoccupation of modern scientists. In the past, humoral theory satisfactorily explained all the manifestations of disease. Physicians turned their attention to grand classifications rather than the minutiae of physiological mechanisms. Gout offered a bountiful terrain for venturesome theoreticians.

"The Tyranny of the Gout"

Along with physicians before him and after, Sydenham put gout into two main categories. First, "regular" gout, which attacks the joints and represents what would today still be considered true gout. Second was the "irregular" gout. The terms used to describe nonarticular gout were as numerous as the symptoms they denoted; most common were irregular, visceral, anomalous, retrocedent, misplaced, atonic, and atopic gout.

Nonarticular disease was accepted as gout if it satisfied the sole criterion of occurring in an individual already labeled "gouty." Consequently, few conditions escaped this category. By the same token, all symptoms in a gouty patient were called "gout." It required little imagination to decide that the nonarticular manifestations might occur in a patient totally lacking the articular symptoms. It was presumed that a patient with, for example, gout pleurisy would have articular gout sometime in the future.

In 1694 William Atkins explained the complexity of gout as follows (21):

> But some have it not in the Joints at all, but in the inward Parts only: and usually when it is in the inward Parts, the Pain is exceeding great for a short time, and runneth about like a Cholick or Spleen, sometimes like the Pain of the Stone, and sometimes like the Gripes in the Bowels, and sometimes like Plurisies. Thus many are afflicted with the Gout of the inward Parts only (p. 6).

This all-encompassing view of irregular gout required additional terms. Alternating, asthenic, flying, larval, masked, latent, repelled, nervous, abarticular, wandering, primitive, and imperfect are but a sampling of the array of modifiers conjoined to "gout" (407, 659). The proliferation of terms was inversely proportional to their content of useful information. None of these conditions persist in modern gout terminology.

In the absence of specific diagnostic criteria, gout could not be separated from other internal diseases. It was believed to move from place to place in the body with an assertive perversity of its own. In its malevolence, gout struck with equal fury the stomach and the kidneys (648). "The gouty Cause often leaves the Joints of the Limbs, and marches up into the Trunk of the Body, where it often settles in the Kidneys, Stomach, or Bowels; or else flies up to the Head, Breast and Lungs, and there mimics the Diseases those respective Parts are subject to" (p. 94).

While George Baker reported to the College of Physicians on Devonshire colic, his contemporaries remained preoccupied writing treatises on gout. In 1767, the gouty vicar of Westham, Ferdinando Warner, published the following passages (779):

> This Gout in the Stomach afflicts Old People most; however, Young People often have it, probably from the Carelessness and Licentiousness in point of Diet. . . .
>
> The Arthritis Collick is very frequent and extremely painful. . . .
>
> Amongst the internal Causes may also be reckoned the Eating and Drinking of improper things; as Fruit or sharp Cyder in too great Quantities or any other Error in point of Ailment, especially those which are of a cold Nature. This Arthritis Collick is often fatal, and always dangerous (pp. 72–76).
>
> It must be allowed that in the Cyder Counties, the Gout is fre-

quent enough to countenance an Opinion that it is in some measure owing to that Liquor (p. 109).

The dominance of abdominal symptoms among the nonarticular manifestations of gout was common knowledge. George Wallis in his notes to Sydenham's *A Treatise of the Gout* attests that, "The paroxysms of the disease are commonly preceded by an affection of the stomach; many of the exciting causes act first upon the stomach; and the atonic and retrocedent gout are most commonly and chiefly affections of the same organ." (723, p. 181).

Warner noted not only the association of gout with colic but recognized encephalopathy as part of the syndrome. He was particularly suspicious of Portugese wines.

> The Portugal, the Spanish and Madeira Wines are too Inflammatory, and contain a great deal of Earthy Matter which creates the Gout: and it is accordingly very observable, that this Distemper hath increased Ten Fold in England, since these Wines have been the Liquor, so much in Use at our Common Tables, and in Taverns. The French Wines, the Sweet, the Turkey and our homemade Smyrna or Currant Wines are not Inflammatory and will do no injury but from their Quantity (p. 224).

At the time that Baker was convincing the College of Physicians that lead caused the Devonshire colic, Warner was describing the association of gout with colic and brain damage. Depicted by William Thackeray as the very model of a fawning courtier, the vicar and his insights were never taken very seriously (743). The failure to recognize acute articular gout as a unique disease is often attributed to the tradition of humoral pathology: observation was submerged by the weight of tradition. It seems possible, however, that the descriptions of irregular gout, rather than distorting daily experience, may have merely reflected clinical encounters with saturnine gout.

The ineffectiveness of available therapy led, over the millennia, to a plethora of innovative remedies. Among the hundreds recorded by Pliny, human urine was neither the most repellent nor the most fanciful. "Man's urine is much commended for the gout in the feet," wrote the Roman chronicler, "as wee may see by Fullers [felt makers] who neuer be goutie, because ordinarily their feet are in men's urine" (607, p. 306). Before the humors lost their claim as the cause of gout, colic and palsy, concoctions including lead were sometimes employed to promote a "cure" (43, 150,

583). In 1653 Riverius included in an extensive catalogue of remedies for gout the following suggestions (644):

> Sal saturni, that is, Salt of Lead, dissolved in subtil Spirit of Wine, easeth pains wonderfully. Frog-spawn-Water stilled in May, applied to the parts pained, doth wonderfully asswage the pains, and tempers the Inflammation and redness of the part. . . . An Infusion of Litharge made in Vinegar, the Vinegar being a little Evaporated, til it grow sweetish, doth much good to an hot Gout (p. 537).

The use of mercury, too, found many supporters. Esteemed as an effective purgative, this heavy metal enjoyed such popularity that few diseases escaped its virtues. In the sixth century, Alexander of Tralles recommended several mercurial remedies, such as calomel for colic and cinnabar for gout. Advocated as mineral theapy by Paracelsus, mercury was not distinguished from lead until the seventeenth century (311). To alchemists, "mercury" was considered an abstract "philosophical" quality, the supposed primary liquid element common to all metals which made its appearance during misconstrued chemical reactions. Molten lead fit the conception of the "philosophical mercury" until seventeenth-century chemists revised the basic concepts of matter (193).

John Woodall deemed mercury so valuable for a variety of afflictions that he published a poem "In Praise of Quick-Silver or Mercurie," the fourth verse of which reads (817):

> The perfectst cure proceeds from thee
> For Pox, for Gout, for Leprosie,
> For Scabs, for Itch, of any Sort,
> These Cures with thee are but a Sport.
>
> (p. 639)

Despite testimonials over many centuries, until recently the value of mercury as an internal therapeutic agent had not been convincingly demonstrated in any human disease (311). Although Boerhaave had noted a striking diuretic response to unspecified mercurial preparations in the seventeenth century (471), quantitative evidence of this response was not recorded until the late nineteenth century (311, 345, 401).

In selecting treatment for gout, accommodation of medical theory took precedence over providing relief. Caverhill recommended that oiled silk be placed on the painful foot which would increase the pain and thereby benefit the gout. If this obnoxious treatment provided insufficient, burning of the flesh over the acutely inflamed joint with moxa was recommended. This ancient oriental torture, introduced to Europe in 1675 by Buxtoff (673) received glowing testimonials from William Temple (737) and was advocated by Boerhaave (77). The ultimate counter-irritation, devised in India, was passed on to eighteenth-century England as straightforward mutilation (122).

> The moxa, or down of mugwort, is applied in the form of a cone, with its base to the part where the pain first begins in the gout. The moxa is fired at the top, and gradually burns down to the skin. The skin is cauterized; but if the pain of the gout is not taken off by the first incineration, the burning is to be renewed to the fourth time, or till the arthritic pain is removed, and the person can set his foot boldly to the ground (p. 141).

Neither the implausibility nor the repugnance of the moxa diminished its popularity. Like tonsillectomy and hysterectomy more recently, to omit the supposed remedy, advocated by laymen and physicians alike, was to invite universal rebuke. To the afflicted, gout and fire were inseparable. The excruciating experience sometimes provoked phlogistic fantasies (21).

> In some the immediate Cause is a hot Vapour or Steam, driven into the parts by the heat of the Blood; and when the Pores are opened where the pain is, this Vapour doth come out like the Smoak of a Chimney, that shall be seen to fill a Room almost with Smoak; and when this Smoak is come out, the pain is presently gone (p. 10).

The author of this passage, William Atkins, claimed "miraculous cures" in addition to metaphysical insight. Sensitive to his background as a self-trained and self-proclaimed "gout doctor," he protests against accusations of sorcery: "When as several say (by reason of the Speediness of my Cures) I use Magick, or the Black Art, to do these things . . . In answer to this I do declare, I have never seen any Books of Astrology" (p. 115).

To William Stukeley and Nicholas Robinson the experience of the gout was incontrovertible evidence of its identity with fire. They envisioned the pain as arising from burning oil (648, 720). Pathophysiology merged with popular imagery as Gillray's *The Gout* (fig. 15) became the essence of the agony (fig. 29). To step from the devil into the fire was second nature to the gouty. Whether the fiery pain was inherent or self-inflicted, the experience was the same (figs. 30–31).

Many of the more prominent symptoms of irregular gout are, in retro-

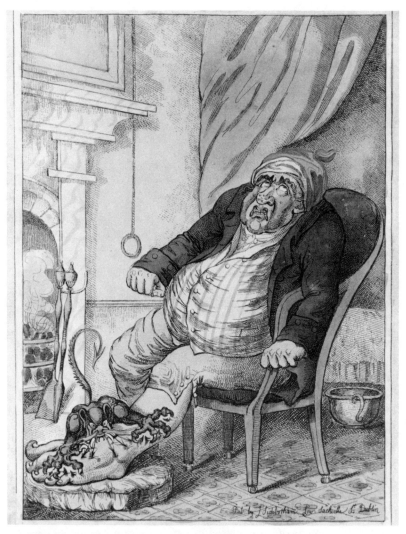

29. The Gout. *Expanding on Gillray's imagery, this fiery podagrical attack engraved by L. S. Low was published about 1800 in Dublin. The bandage on the head, common in gout caricatures, suggests the systemic nature of the disease in its "irregular" form. From the author's collection.*

spect, more reasonably attributed to lead poisoning: colic, palsy, brain disorders, and convulsions. But the possibility that these symptoms might be due to lead seems never to have been entertained. Physicians were more inclined to spread the lore of their teachers. Metaphors for irregular gout remained exuberant as the twentieth century approached.

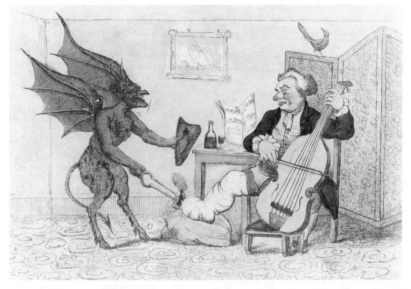

30. The Origin of the Gout *was the Devil, fire, and the discriminating taste of the intellectual dilettante. Engraved by W. H. Bunbury in 1785. From the collection of the National Library of Medicine.*

"Suppressed or undeveloped gout," wrote J. Mortimer Granville in 1881, "is like the subterranean operation of volcanic forces, the attack being the earthquake or eruption, with an outpouring of lava" (326, p. 575).

While "irregular gout" was never specifically rejected, the term gradually fell into disuse. With refinements of classification, clinical connections between wine, gout, lead, and the kidney were lost. In the colonial period, however, traditional views prevailed.

In prerevolutionary America rum was the favored drink. Whether it was imported from Jamaica or from New England, lead poisoning from this popular repast was common. Franklin and Cadwalader appreciated some of the dangers of rum, but neither included gout among its legacies. Benjamin Rush, physician signatory of the Declaration of Independence, saw gout as one of the many evil consequences of Demon Rum. To him the injury was more moral than physical. In 1774, America's most revered physician presented a rousing public attack on drinking and tyranny to the Philosophical Society of Philadelphia (661).

> I have heard of two or three cases of GOUT among the Indians, but it was only those who had learned the use of rum from the white people. . . . The effects of wine, like tyranny in a well formed

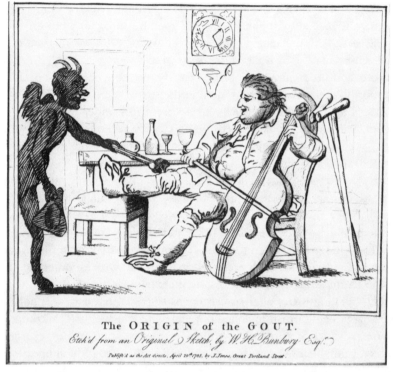

The ORIGIN of the GOUT.
Etch'd from an Original Sketch, by W. H. Bunbury Esq.

Publish'd as the Act directs, April 20th 1785, by J. Jones, Great Portland Street.

31. Bunbury's insight (fig. 30) struck a popular chord and was copied in the same year, 1785, in an engraving by J. Jones. From the author's collection.

government, are felt first in the extremities; while spirits, like a bold invader, seize at once upon the vitals of the constitution (pp. 263–64).

While Rush did not suspect lead in the rum, in his temperance tract on "Inquiry into the Effects of Ardent Spirits upon the Human Body," he included among the evil consequences of liquor, "gout in all its various forms of swelled limbs, colic, palsy and apoplexy" (661, p. 157)—a concise description of saturnism.

Resisting the prodigious proliferation of disease entities espoused by his teacher William Cullen, Rush swung to doctrinaire oversimplification, to the Brunonian system of medicine, a fashionable way of thinking about the materia medica which caused a sudden, if temporary, decline in medical progress and soon became the focus of bitter satire (99).

Ignoring contemporary advances in chemistry and lacking any systematic approach to etiologic diagnosis, Rush came to believe that all manifestations of disease were, in fact, merely different aspects of a single phe-nomenon. Baffled by the many faces of gout, he opted for a unitary view of disease. With unflagging confidence he wrote, "However varied mor-bid actions may be by their causes, seats, and effects, they are all the same nature, and the time will probably come when the whole nomenclature of morbid actions will be absorbed in the single name of disease" (661, p. 234). Rush included virtually all disease states under the heading of "gout." "In short," he explained, "the gout may be compared to a mon-arch whose empire is unlimited. The whole body crouches before it" (p. 250).

In 1811 Rush edited an American edition of Hillary. But despite his friendship with Benjamin Franklin, William Currie, and Thomas Cadwalader, men with an intimate knowledge of colica Pictonum, Amer-ica's most renowned physician never perceived a connection between lead and the protean manifestations of gout. Consistent with the Bruno-nian view of disease, Rush preferred to treat gout with bloodletting, just as he treated other illnesses. Despite great faith in this method of treat-ment, his long list of alternate regimens suggests that cure was not the invariable result. Rush included purging, emetic, nitre, cold, warmth, li-quors, abstinence, turpentine, blisters, terror, sweating, opium, exercise, moxa, calomel and a variety of herbs, vegetables, and local applications.

An astute politician, brilliant conversationalist, but questionable practi-tioner, Rush developed ponderous theories of physic. His reputation as a patriot was eventually eclipsed by his disastrous medical practice, since, at his hands, Americans bled as profusely for "cure" as ever they had for liberty. In his later years, Rush lost faith in the efficacy of phlebotomy, but managed to do equal damage with mercury (742).

Rush did not eschew political influence to silence his critics. One self-proclaimed gadfly, William Cobbett, was forced to flee Philadelphia, his belongings confiscated by court order, for attacking Rush's system of medicine. Cobbett continued to fling barbs at phlebotomy and calomel from New York in his *Porcupine's Gazette*. Cobbett "could not be per-suaded that 'bleeding almost to death' was likely to save life" (147). Un-der the pen name, Peter Porcupine, he advised his readers that at the very moment the court sentenced him for libeling Rush, George Washington was dying at the hands of adherents to Rush's System of Medicine. From news reports Cobbett calculated that no less than 108 ounces were bled from the Father of Our Country during the last twenty hours of his life.

Rush reserved lead for the treatment of epilepsy in children. Reporting this therapy in 1804, he revealed the basis of his remarkable discovery

(660). "I was first led to prescribe sugar of lead in epilepsy, by hearing that a man had been cured of it, by swallowing part of a table spoonful of white lead by mistake, instead of a table spoonful of loaf sugar." Dr. Thomas R. P. Spence of Virginia paid homage to Rush in 1806 when reporting the successful cure of his own epilepsy by the use of lead. Spence consumed enough sugar of lead to incur severe colic (698). His seizures did not recur and he therefore believed that he had advanced medical science by extending Rush's pediatric cure to adults. Rush's medical bag, preserved for posterity at the College of Physicians of Philadelphia, contains a vial of Extract of Lead ready for the next house call.

The *Inaugural Dissertation* of one of his students affords a dismal view of the medical arts in Philadelphia in the wake of the famed teacher. William Webb, writing in 1798, attempted to mold George Baker's findings into the unitary theory of Rush with the following results (783):

> There is but one remote cause of fever * (*Vido Dr. Rush's Inquiries, vol. 4, p. 132); and there is but one remote cause of colic, and that is stimulous. Heat alternating with cold, marsh miasmata; the fumes of lead and other poisons; passions of the mind, and the like, all act by stimulating power producing colic. Hence it is that the symptoms of the colic are the same, differing only in degree although the causes which produce them are innumerable.
>
> The paralysis of the extremities, in colic, has mostly been ascribed to the effects of lead; but this effect can only be produced from the excessive force of stimulous, as the length of time for which it is applied; this appears clearly from its being produced from other causes than that of lead (p. 17).

Young Dr. Webb went on to group intestinal obstruction, biliary obstruction, paralytic ileus, cholera, dysentery, and indeed the full spectrum of intestinal diseases as a single ailment. Not surprisingly he was confident that, "the most judicious method of curing the colic, is first to diminish the excitement by blood-letting" (p. 23). "I shall ever lament the death," he confessed, "of a young man, who was affected with the colic, and whose friends persuaded him against the use of the lancet; . . . he died for want of more bleeding!" (p. 22). Mercury, he averred, was a good second choice to cure the colic. Undoubtedly his professor, Benjamin Rush, commended Dr. Webb for having learned his lessons well. While Oliver Wendell Holmes could announce the passing of venesection from American medical practice in 1861, twenty years later it was still popular among physicians under Rush's influence in New Jersey (163).

Rich in the rationalism of the times, eighteenth-century medicine was impoverished of common sense. Systems of medicine designed to account for a vast spectrum of vaguely formulated biologic phenomena collapsed under the burden of fanciful theories and testimonials. Paying homage to science, the leading academicians preached biologic truth with theologic fervor. Incomprehensible gibberish discouraged even the most scholarly. In the past, as in the present, the influence of physicians was often determined as much by their charm as by their insight. Scholarship was sometimes judged more by verbosity than quality, but eminence was no guarantor of competence.

Unsupported conclusions from unbridled speculation were by no means limited to the eighteenth century. While introducing chemical enlightenment to clinical practice, Henry Bence-Jones also popularized the view that uric acid was poisonous, especially to the kidneys (61, p. 134). The idea that uric acid contaminated the blood conjured up feelings of horror in the public mind in the twentieth century too. Patent medicine entrepreneurs capitalized on the terror of the insidious kidney poison by purveying cures for the detestable waste product. De Witt's Kidney & Bladder Pills promised to remove the "fetid matter" from those whose lives it might cut short (fig. 32). The threat of uric acid to the kidneys remained a selling point for allopurinol in 1982 (fig. 33).

According to Alexander Haig in *Uric Acid as a Factor in the Causation of Disease*, gout was the cause of lead colic (345). "Lead colic," Haig stated, "is simply an enteralgia or enteritis, produced by the irritant effects of urate of lead in the intestinal walls" (p. 403). In an attempt to reconcile incompatible views of gout, Haig revived "irregular gout" by arguing that a wide range of diseases were caused by urate deposition. Espousing a unitary hypothesis reminiscent of Rush, he included in addition to gout, a host of unrelated conditions which he believed were caused by hyperuricemia: migraine, epilepsy, hysteria, mental disease, syncope, asthma, bronchitis, dyspepsia, colic, Raynaud's disease, paroxysmal hemoglobinuria, anemia, Bright's disease, diabetes mellitus, rheumatoid arthritis, and rheumatic heart disease. The ability to measure uric acid in blood did not guarantee a more reasonable approach to the classification of gout.

The abundance of absurdity in the treatment of gout did not pass unnoticed by its victims. An emerging literary subculture vented frustration with direct attacks on the "gout doctors." Few diseases did more to denigrate the already doubtful reputation of physicians. Alluding to the intransigence of gout, we have from the "councils" of the great sixteenth-

Are You Poisoned?

IS YOUR SYSTEM SATURATED WITH DEADLY, INSIDIOUS URIC ACID?

If so, you are only one of the many thousands whose lives are made miserable by this most malignant poison.

Uric acid in the system is a product of the waste matter in the blood which is not properly filtered and removed by the kidneys.

It is the duty of these important organs to remove this poisonous and fetid matter from the blood and dispose of it as Nature intended, and when they fail to do so, the character of this product rapidly changes until there is produced in the blood a virulent and malignant poison.

This is Uric Acid and it has a deleterious effect upon every organ, bone and sinew of the body, and its ravages are indicated by the excruciating pains of Rheumatism, Backache, and all the other well-known symptoms.

Now, you know what Uric Acid is—why it exists—the ills it produces, and you naturally inquire how can it be removed, and what shall be used for the purpose.

The answer plainly is—keep the kidneys in condition to remove the poisonous acid from your system as fast as it accumulates.

For this purpose, we recommend **DeWitt's Kidney & Bladder Pills.** They have a world-wide reputation for efficiency in checking kidney and bladder troubles, and thousands of sufferers in this country testify to the relief they have given them. Your druggist should be able to supply you with either the 50c trial size or the $1.00 family size. If not, send us the price and we will forward them at once prepaid. **Ingredients can be imitated but not our years of experience in making** **"DeWitt's"** reliable preparations.

32. Fear of "deadly, insidious uric acid" stimulated sales of Dewitt's Kidney & Bladder Pills, at the turn of the century. From the author's collection.

century physician John Fernel, the following (644): "And at length, if it be let alone, it grows into an incurable stoney hardness of which the Poet [says] 'when gouty Humors into stones convert, they jeere the Doctors, and despise their Art'" (p. 334). In 1737 John Marten recorded similar dismay (515): "All th' Art of Physick cannot rout / The Stubborn Pains of Knotty Gout" (p. 47). A watercolor by G. M. Woodward of 1798 illustrates the layman's pervasive sense of betrayal by physicians. A gout-ridden doctor carouses with the devil while his comrade, an undertaker, shares his pleasures with death himself (fig. 34). This particular image

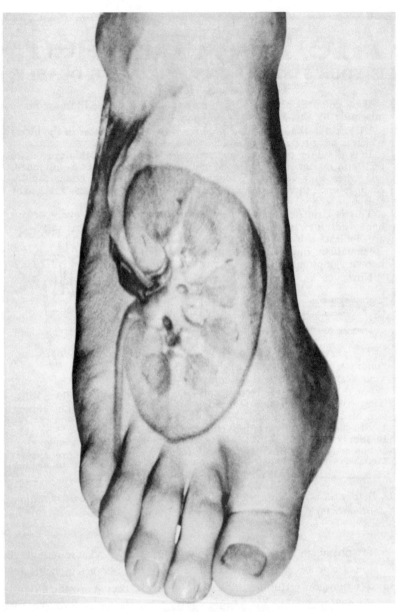

33. In 1982, fear of the nephrotoxic effect of uric acid stimulated the sales of allopurinol as seen in this illustration for an advertisement for Zyloprim. By permission of Burroughs Wellcome Co.

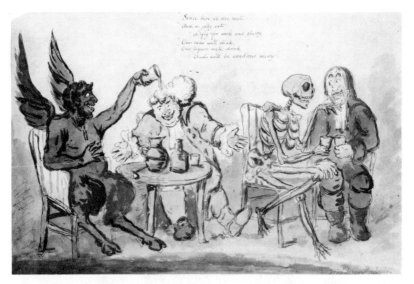

34. In the Doctor and His Friends, *a watercolor painted by G. M. Woodward in 1798, we see that the Devil, Death and the gout are the Doctor's constant drinking companions. From the Philadelphia Museum of Art: SmithKline Corporation Collection.*

gained wide circulation in a copy etched by Isaac Cruikshank in the same year.

Following traditions traced to the fourteenth century, quacks abounded in seventeenth-century London (747). Taking their cues from the learned in physic, the distinctions between pretense and legitimacy were more a matter of style than substance. Renegade practitioners outdid academe with showmanship graced with the trappings of scholarship. Latin, Greek, and literary gifts were the stock-in trade of the peddlers of cures. Nor was their appeal limited to the ignorant and lowly. John Pechey, William Salmon, and John Hill, among the most prosperous of London's quacks, were prolific and erudite writers whose works were coveted by the gentry as well as by the masses. Royal occultists, as well as royal physicians, counseled the king to assure His Majesty of balanced advice. Scoundrels mimicked the learned faculty, and poets parodied the quacks. The "Infallible Mountebank," proclaimed (747):

> See Sirs, See here (he cries)
> A Doctor rare
> Who travels much at home,
> Here take my bills,

I cure all ills,
Past, Present and to Come,
The Cramp, the Stitch,
The Squirt, the Itch,
The Gout, the Stone, the Pox,
The Mulligrubs,
The Bonny Scrubs,
And all Pandora's Box,
Thousands I've Dissected,
Thousands new erected,
And such Cures effected,
As none ere can tell,
Let the Palsie shake ye,
Let the Crinkums break ye,
Let Murrain take ye;
Take this, and you are well.

(p. 77)

Whether this broadside was directed at the true or counterfeit physicians was not at all clear.

Lack of agreement on the nature of the disease made it equally difficult to agree upon a cure. Pathophysiology remained an art, born of experience and intuition, rather than rigorous analysis. Traditional concepts of etiology elicited as much condemnation as did useless remedies. Richard Blackmore discounted venery as a cause of gout (72) on strictly logical grounds while John Floyer leaped to its defense (262).

So lay the Load upon the right Horse, and Saddle old Bacchus's Back, as the chief Author and Contriver of this Joint-Evil, and ask Venus Pardon for laying a drunken Brat at her Door, which she never deserv'd;
And this it is, to be ill nam'd,
When a poor Whore is (wrongly) blam'd.

(p. 368)

Physicians found themselves in a defensive posture. Their strained logic was not persuasive. "A person must have the Gout, or suffer much worse," wrote John Quincy. "And it is the Duty and Business of Medicine to forward and procure this Tormentor, rather than pretend to prevent, or cure it. . . . What must we then think of the Tribe of Empirics," he expounded, "who are continually stuffing the daily Papers with Advertisements and Pretensions of Cure in this Case, but that they are a Drove of Robbers and Murtherers" (615, p. 434). The competition for recognition was ferocious; no holds were barred. In the past, fraud in medical practice elicited outrage that today is found only in condemnations of fraud in research.

Few gout doctors provoked more ridicule than Robert Kinglake. Discounting the idea of a "morbific matter" and rejecting the concept of displacement, Kinglake insisted that the disease was purely a local phenomenon, analogous to a sprain—a consequence of excessive excitability of the ligaments (420). He promised cure of the gout by local application of cold water. "It should not be forgotten," he explained, "that the object to be effected is literally the extinction of fire" (p. 84). His pretentious proposal of what was largely common sense won the wrath of a public primed for more elegant doctrines.

Kinglake reveled in the attention won by his controversial "refrigerant" treatment. Comparing his contribution with that of Harvey and Jenner, Dr. Kinglake reproduced in his book, among many favorable testimonials, two which heaped scorn rather than approbation upon himself. "What in truth moved my bile," wrote one anonymous critic, "was the pompous manner in which Dr. K announced the application of cold water in gout, as a novel practice originating with himself; and for which he seemed hastily to elicit applause due to a public benefactor" (p. 278). To such thrusts Kinglake responded in footnotes, without recourse to modesty, "Your shaft reached, not its mark, it fell harmless before the shrine of truth, and served the useful purpose of proclaiming your forfeiture of all future credibility" (p. 288). One "author of Historical Surgery," J. Hunt, appraised Kinglake's work as follows (387):

> The first case which Dr. Kinglake has brought forward in behalf of his favourite hypothesis, most evidently displays the inaccuracy of his observation; and the pains that he has taken to complete the accommodation with the bombastic language he has made use of, expose beyond all doubt the cloud of misrepresentation which was intended to disguise the light of truth (p. 38).

Not content with this chastisement, Hunt went on to appraise the Brunonian system from which Kinglake gained inspiration.

> The Brunonian system: in the most advantageous point of view, can only be considered as a theory of health; for as the Author had no practice, it was impossible he should have had the least knowl-

edge of disease; except we suppose that, as he was himself a martyr to intemperance and the gout, the operations of his own constitution formed the basis on which the Elementa Medicinae was first established. And even under these circumstances we do not meet with a coincidence of opinion: for though Dr. Kinglake's book exhibits a most accomplished example of Brunonian insanity, yet on the subject of gout these great Doctors do not agree in a single instance, either in theory or practice (p. 82).

Kinglake's "principles of common sense" also drew fire from professional colleagues. In 1805 William Perry published nine mythical dialogues entitled *A dialogue in the Shades, Recommended to Every Purchaser of Dr. Kinglake's Dissertation, &c., as an Appropriate Tailpiece for Embellishment and Illustrations by Sir John Floyer's Ghost.* The scenario has Mercury ferrying the ghosts of victims across the River Styx. Each applicant for entry to Elysium is questioned by Mercury as, for example, a naval captain (599):

Mercury.
I see your former sufferings, Captain, have been great. Where was that leg lost?
Captain.
Under Howe in the fight of June 1st.
Mercury.
What has ended your career of Honour at last?
Captain.
Possibly, Mercury, the best short answer would be Gout. But a comparison of the last experiment with former modes of relief, bids me add—"The cooperation of Cold Water, within and without."
Mercury.
You seem to speak of Water having a full trial, if not a fair one. Was this your first fit?
Captain.
No,—I had many attacks in the last ten years.
The Surgeon of the Ship I have now left thought to cure me speedily by a new method.
Mercury.
Of his own, or recommended?
Captain.

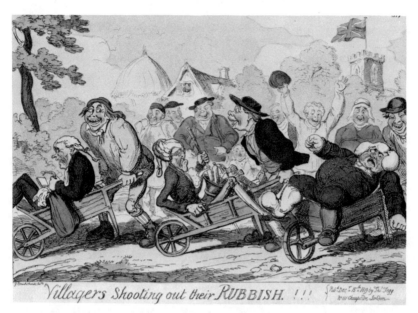

35. Villagers Shooting out their Rubbish, *engraving by George Cruikshank, 1819. The garbage includes a barrister, an apothecary (doctor?) with patent medicines, and a rotund, gouty pastor. From the author's collection.*

Recommended by a West Country Physician. Dr. Kin—— Kin—— Killkin or some such ugly name. Prior to this finishing stroke, I had always parried affections of the Stomach by Madeira or by Brandy; but was unluckily through our Surgeon's confidence in this new method dissuaded from my customary remedies. Two days or less settled the account, and I am at this moment quite of opinion—that not "Gout," but "Water" brought my years of Warfare to an end.

(Dialogue V, pp. 30—32)

The scorn of "gout doctors" was portrayed by George Cruikshank in a caricature entitled *Villagers Shooting out their Rubbish.* The central figure is an apothecary (or, perhaps, doctor with gold-headed cane) surrounded by a gouty pastor (on the right) and attorney (on the left), all dispatched to the village dump (fig. 35). "Good-by, Doctor!" proclaimed an ad for Perry Davis' Vegetable Pain Killer some one hundred and fifty years later (fig. 36).

The bottle was, perhaps better solace for the gout than was the medi-

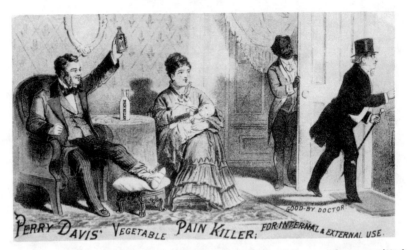

36. Perry Davis' Vegetable Pain Killer not only relieved the gout but permitted the patient to bid "Good-by, Doctor!" Chromolithograph trade card, about 1890. From the author's collection.

cal doctor. The patent medicine was guaranteed to cure the colic as well as the gout.

In 1699, with mordant irony Philander Misaurius (pseudonym) dedicated to all physicians *The Honour of the Gout* (530). In the introduction Philander states his harsh view of physicians.

> This is certain, like true Farriers, you have prescribed to many a meak man a medicine for a horse. So then for the Materia Medica 'tis the same. Nothing be troublesome and uneasy to you in your new Profession, but that you shall never get as much by practicing on the Spavin as the Gout: but you must content yourself with less earnings. What! You can't in conscience expect as much for killing a Horse as a Man (p. ii).

Finding a kindred spirit in wit and wisdom, Benjamin Franklin reprinted this satirical piece in Philadelphia in 1732. Some five decades later, having endured the gout himself, Franklin wrote *A Dialogue with the Gout*. Like many a fine physician, Franklin had little use for professionals when his own illness was at issue. Discoursing with Gout personified, Franklin strove to keep his enemy talking, lest Gout exercise his painful office (270).

Franklin: Ah! how tiresome you are!

Gout: Well, then, to my office: it should not be forgotten that I am your physician. There!

Franklin: Oh-h-h! What a devil of a physician!

Gout: How ungrateful you are to say so! Is it not I, who, in the character of your physician, have saved you from the palsy, dropsy and apoplexy? one or other of which would have done for you long ago but for me.

Franklin: I submit and thank you for the past, but entreat the discontinuance of your visits for the future: for in my mind one had better die than be cured so dolefully. Permit me just to hint that I have also not been unfriendly to you. I never feed physician or quack of any kind to enter the list against you; if then, you do not leave me to my repose, it may be said you are ungrateful too.

Gout: I can scarcely acknowledge that as an objection. As to quacks, I despise them: they may kill you indeed, but cannot injure me. And as to regular physicians, they are at last convinced that the gout, in such a subject as you are, is no disease, but a remedy; and wherefore cure a remedy?

Always the self-reliant individualist, Franklin is said to have discovered Husson's secret remedy and imported it to America (729).

As is not infrequently the case, doctors were often their own worst enemies. Touting a series of useless remedies, they paused only long enough to ridicule their competitors' choice. Pushing his own wonder drug, muriatic acid (hydrochloric), William Rowley roundly attacked the traditional milk-cure (659). Rejecting abstinence in all its forms, Rowley conceded that milk was occasionally harmless. "In other instances," he complained, "a dropsy has been the consequence, which has cured the gout, but killed the patient" (p. 40). Rowley believed that since muriatic acid could crystallize "the calcerous matter" (uric acid) out of solutions, it would similarly draw it out of the joints when applied to the skin.

R. Drake, a disgruntled London apothecary, explained why he was so eager to sell his own secret cure (201).

The end I propose in publishing this essay is, to lay before the candid and impartial reader, a plain, succinct history of the conduct of our sage physicians, in this their darling distemper, which they are pleased to term "a friend to long life," though the scandal of physic, but the Diana by which they accumulate great wealth: . . .

It is a truth too obvious, that our physical gentry have not advanced one step towards this lucky discovery; and since the days of Hippocrates have been blundering on, in their old beaten road and track, in ignorance and bare-faced error (pp. 1–2).

Drake crossed the fine line between wisdom and quackery with a facility born of righteous indignation goaded by greed. His specific for gout consisted of flowers, herbs, roots and seeds; "a very large collection, and as numerous as any medicine which the dispensatory directs" (p. 30). He recommended his remedy as a pleasant medicine which, in contrast to the harsh remedies of his physician adversaries, made people feel better.

The apothecary promised to comfort his patients, not to increase their suffering. He urged them to drink a pint of Madeira, rum, or brandy punch an hour after taking his secret concoction. Alternating homely advice with aggressive assault, he railed against contemptible physicians (201).

> How extremely preposterous and whimsical in our medical-gentry, is their debarring the thirsty Arthritic the total relish of that most grateful, most comfortable fluid, punch? . . . Until such time as these adepts in physic recant their errors, and assign a more rational and convincing reason for their singular but shuffling prohibition of it, I shall continue affirming it to be the most salubrious liquor, for all such as are subject to this painful malady (pp. 32–33).

Drake's rancor was at times eloquent.

> This great city will never be without vain pretenders to the cure of diseases, for where there is honey will also be flies; and the great number of Arthritics which our luxurious manner of living produces, intitle us to swarms of these locusts from all parts of the globe (p. 49).

At other times he seemed defensive.

> If you enquire of these physical oracles what the Gout is, they give you an ambiguous and obscure answer, say it is something which falls on the joints; but what that something is, you are to fathom and discover. Pray then, what are these wise men about? eating up the people as if they were bread? I answer, only picking your pockets a-la-mode. So great are their infatuations, that they know not how to treat the Gout, or administer the least relief; yet can rail, with great freedom, at Quacks and Pretenders to cure the Gout, at

the same time that they are nothing but Quacks and Pretenders themselves. . . .

. . . Indeed, there is one Drake, a man in private life, and much beneath their notice; who has some of the spirit of quackerism in him, a specific for the Gout, and for the Dropsy. If these are considered in that light, and qualify him for that honourable appellation, then all are quacks indeed (pp. 67–69).

But in an earlier *Essay on the Nature and Method of Treating the Gout* published in 1751, Drake noted in a postscript some reservations about adulterated Madeira (200). "P.S. Arthritics in the Country express the great Difficulty which attends procuring genuine Madeira Wine, and say, what is sold for Madeira, is a most wretched, sour, and corrupt Mixture or Wine, which disorders the Stomach, creates an unusual Heat like Brandy and frequently gripes" (p. 71). Despite his venomous judgements, Drake came very close to the mark well before Baker. He rejected the "acid salts" hypothesis and suspected that contaminants in Madeira were responsible for the gout.

William Cadogen's assertion that "gout be the necessary effect of intemperance" aroused particular contempt (63, 250, 689). One anonymous author's vilification of Cadogen grew intemperate (250).

Some persons will deem it ingratitude in you, Doctor, to rail against the luxuries of the table, wine, music, women, &c. which from the complaints you have exhibited to the world, you seem to have enjoyed with an extraordinary and uncommon gout, with the most soft and pleasing delight, even with rapture. I view this behavior in a more favorable, and I trust in a true light. You are now repenting (may Merciful Heaven accept your repentance though late!) of the follies and indiscretions of your juvenile days (pp. 24–25).

"Anonymous" will have none of it! With youthful abandon he decried medical hypocrisy. "For my own part, I will not abstain from any of them, that is pleasing and agreeable to my appetite, yet use them with temperance and moderation, and then only leave them, when I find them hurtful to my constitution and destructive of my health, or like the old Doctor, I can not longer taste or relish them" (p. 36).

William Carter was similarly disenchanted with Cadogen's regimen. In *A Free and Candid Examination of Dr. Cadogen's Dissertation on the Gout*, Carter questioned the value of abstinence (120).

Persons afflicted with the gout are generally joyous; love their bottle and their friend, and to take them off intirely from wine, must be a penance, few or none, will submit to (p. 12).

Tho' the Doctor has painted, in most lively colours the mischiefs arising from intemperance, he seems to have carried matters a little too far, in recommending to us a journey to Spain, Portugal or Italy, to learn temperance. This is enjoining a penance, which no free-born Englishman, I apprehend, will submit to (p. 27).

The Doctor Dissected or Willy Cadogen in the Kitchen. Addressed to all Invalids and Readers of a late Dissertation on the gout &c, &c, &c. was published anonymously "By a Lady" in 1771. The title page assures us "The best of all Doctors is sweet Willy O." The parody alternately paraphrases and knifes Dr. Cadogen (433).

> The gout, a disease now so common has grown,
> That scarce lives a man, but its twinges have known;
> Or, say he show'd not, full as well explain,
> Its cause, and its several stages of pain:
> Unless to the stomach, it chance to get clear in,
> And then he'll pronounce you, dead as a herring
>
> (p. 3)

The final verse thrusts home, reciting a perennial view of physicians that never loses its sting.

> Adieu! to the practice of doctors elect:
> You'd best then, remain Sirs, *aut Caesar, aux Nullus*,
> Of our money and lives, with formality, cull us;
> Nay, I'll not mince the matter,—in troth I hate lying.
> "In Minimis" take it—you live by our dying.
>
> (p. 21)

Practitioners found themselves emphasizing the brighter side of the affliction; gout was a mark of distinction. Robinson recalled the glory of the grand debauchee (648).

We find, by dear-bought Experience, that this Disease most commonly attacks those Persons, upon the Decline of Life, that, in their younger Years, have spent their Time in too liberal Use of Wine, Women and a salacious Diet; that is, that have drank deep in the fashionable Vices of the Age we live in. The Persons most inclinable to suffer under the Tyranny of the Gout, . . . are generally those that have large Heads, great Hearts, and strong Passions; and who, most commonly, are Men of Genius, Spirit, and Courage (p. 34).

Ridicule naturally pursued such arrogance. Scorn rather than empathy was evident in the caricatures of Gillray, Rowlandson, and Cruikshank. The victims of the gout were frequently the least compassionate. Even "Mother Goose" was pitiless in warning the nursery of the wrath of a vengeful father (658).

> Lazy Tom with jacket blue,
> Stole his father's gouty shoe,
> The worst of harm that Dad can wish him,
> Is his gouty shoe may fit him.

The Age of Reason contributed little more than the Age of Mysticism to the solution of the mysteries of gout. Ideas of causation remained as ambiguous as ever. Frustration was vented on the proponents of humoral theory and abstinence. Real progress in understanding etiology could only be made through the application of chemistry to medicine. Anatomic pathology of the nineteenth century had to displace the moral philosophy of the eighteenth. Measurements of uric acid provided a more limited definition of gout and eventually a basis for treatment. In time, physicians no longer felt compelled to attribute all the ills of mankind to the gouty diathesis. By common consent, gout became a specific arthritic complaint rather than a systemic disease. Only one vital internal organ, the kidney, remained subject to its attack. Renal disease survives as the one serious manifestation of nonarticular gout. More mysteries dwelled in the urine than even the most ardent watercaster supposed (fig. 37).

Saturnine Gout

The role of lead in causing gout was all but ignored until the work of A. B. Garrod, largely because neither George Baker nor Tanquerel des Planches mentioned it. Baker's omission of saturnine gout was not an oversight. In accord with eighteenth-century thinking, he considered irregular gout a distinct affliction of the viscera (34).

> But, although it be not denied, that the gout and the rheumatism do sometimes quit their proper station, and attack the stomach and intestines; yet experience by no means testifies, that palsy is the ordinary consequence of such an attack. A pain in the bowels, aris-

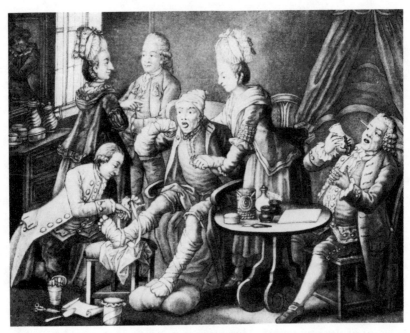

37. *In the eighteenth century, the doctor's visit to* A Podagrical Man *included wrapping the gouty legs and inspection of the urine, as depicted in an engraving by J. Ph. Haid, about 1750. The Devil is found hiding in the uroscopy flask. The Bettmann Archive, Inc.*

ing from a gouty cause, under proper management, generally returns to the extremities; which are very apt, for some time afterwards, to be swollen, and weakened. But a paralytic affection is not the usual termination of an arthritic colic (p. 385).

Physicians had, however, received intimations of the role of lead through a number of isolated observations in the past. Barrough had noted the association of gout with colic in the sixteenth century and Citois made similar observations in the colic of Poitou. Shortly thereafter, Daniel Sennert recognized that "Epidemical gout" was associated "with the Stone, Colick, . . . the Palsie and Contraction of the Members and the Falling-sickness" (679, p. 7). In the Paracelsian tradition, Sennert attributed this symptom complex to the "tartarous matter" of wine. But he viewed "tartar" more as an extraneous contaminant than the nebulous "acid residue" of Paracelsus. "Minerals, Metals and divers kinds of Earth", were, he believed, absorbed by grape vines grown in "Clayish grounds." This "Mineral juyce as it were, and such as is wholly unuseful to our bodies, which is not unfitly termed Tartar . . . [is] by Nature thrust into the Joynts." It

> sticketh fast unto the sides of the Casks, but is likewise, thoroughly mingled with the substance of the Wine. And this is altogether the Nature of the Salts that they reduce other bodies into the Smallest Atomes, and then do associate the Atomes into themselves. We may see an experiment of this in the dissolving of Metals in strong Waters, in which Metals (bodies otherwise thick) are so united into the Salt of the Waters that dissolve them, that they may pass through a Card or Paper (p. 14).

This prophetic analogy between the tartar of wines and the solubilization of metals projected the mineral contaminant as the direct cause of the gout—a role present-day physicians would reserve for uric acid. Moreover, Sennert believed the noxious component was absorbed from the soil rather than added later in the fermentation process.

As we have seen, in 1671 Johann Jacob Wepfer (799) used chemical techniques to demonstrate that lead in wine was the source of many ills, including gout. All the elements of saturnine gout were thus assembled: gout, colic, palsy, and metalic contaminants in wine. But the evidence needed for general acceptance was still incomplete. The saturnine link between wine and gout could only be made after George Baker convinced doctors that lead was the cause of the Devonshire colic.

That lead contributed to the development of gout was recorded by James Hardy, one of Baker's staunchest supporters. Embroiled in the defense of Baker's thesis, Hardy's association of gout with lead was perhaps obscured by his rhetoric (773). In response, "a physician at Newburg," J. Francis Riollay, indignantly denied the culpability of cider. "Permit us, then Sir, without trembling for the consequences," begged Riollay, "to enjoy moderately one of the greatest blessings of life" (642, p. 42). In his polemical retort, Hardy stated his conclusion concerning gout on his title page (fig. 38, [354]): "Gout originates from the Action of Mineral Substances, especially those conveyed into the Human System by the Medium of adulterated Wines." By "Mineral Substances," Hardy meant primarily lead, but he did not exclude the possibility that gypsum, mercury, antimony, zinc, and arsenic might also contribute to gout. He acknowledged that several authors in the past had recognized the constellation of signs and symptoms arising from lead poisoning.

Previous writers, however, had not usually understood the role of adulterants in alcoholic beverages. Apparently unaware of Wepfer's publica-

AN

A N S W E R

TO THE

L E T T E R

ADDRESSED BY

FRANCIS RIOLLAY, ∨

PHYSICIAN OF NEWBURY,

TO

Dr. HARDY, on the Hints given concerning
the Origin of the GOUT, in his Publication
on the COLIC of DEVON;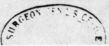

IN WHICH

The several OBJECTIONS made by Dr. RIOLLAY are
considered; and the Probability that the GOUT
originates from the Action of Mineral Substances,
especially those conveyed into the Human System by the
Medium of adulterated Wines, is more fully insisted on,

By JAMES HARDY, M.D. ∕

———————————

L O N D O N:

Printed for T. CADELL, in the Strand; and
RICHARDSON and URQUHART, at the Royal
Exchange.   MDCCLXXX.

*38. The title page of James Hardy's pamphlet of 1780 attributing the gout and
the colic of Devon to the adulteration of wine with lead. From the collection
of the National Library of Medicine.*

tion, Hardy cited the work of Zeller and Weisman in 1707 as the first hints of lead as a cause of gout. Arguing rhetorically he continued:

> Now as we are both agreed and persuaded, that the causes of colic, and the paralytic consequences, are sufficiently demonstrated to have risen from lead, gypsum and arsenic exclusively; have you not Sir, been rather hasty in thus peremptorily passing censure on me, for extending my views to the other disease, whose origin has hitherto been equally inexplicable, and which appears from the writings of most esteemed authors, thus closely connected with them? I submit to your calm reconsideration, if there be not the most rational ground for such an opinion;—and since the gout is not observed to be the crisis of any disease in nature, except this particular species of colic, is it not a matter worthy of our most deliberate enquiry? (p. 47).

Hardy recognized many sources of lead exposure and that gout was not a constant result of poisoning.

> The position I would be understood to have initiated, and from which I wish not to recede, is this, that the primary causes of the gout, so far as at present can be ascertained with any degree of precision, arise from the action of mineral substances admitted into the human system. There are several ways they may gain admission and therefore I by no means consent to be confined to that of adulterated liquors only, though I should readily admit that 17 or 18 out of every 20 gouty cases, have been originally produced by means of such liquors (p. 5).

In contrast to Baker, Hardy gave credence to the earlier observations of Citois, Musgrave, and Huxham concerning gout as a late sequela of colic. But Hardy was only a minor figure in the interminable debates on both lead and gout. Medical opposition to lead-gout had a different tone than the disapprobation that greeted Baker's initial revelation. Silence rather than polemics met Hardy's description of saturnine gout. His assertion of causality was vulnerable to equally arbitrary rebuttal (350).

James Hardy's deductions were widely ignored. Yet, in 1785, William Withering described a case of "irregular gout" due, he "suspected [and proved], to the poison of lead" (815, p. 46). Within the decade, George Wallis recalled that adulterants in wine might be the cause of gout (723) and, in 1807, Caleb Hillier Parry rediscovered the association of lead and gout (588). In both France (128) and England, Parry received credit for the first description of saturnine gout, although his observations followed Wepfer's by a century and a half and Hardy's by a quarter of a century. Parry's writings, published posthumously in 1825, contain a single paragraph on the subject entitled "Gout from Lead" in which he stated, "I observe that after the palsy from lead, patients of a middle age, otherwise previously healthy, are very subject to fits of gout in the limbs" (588, p. 243).

Unaware of earlier contributions to the subject, Garrod claimed priority (289).

> The relationship between lead impregnation and gout was not, I believe, made publically known before 1854, when in a paper read before the Medico-Chirurgical Society, and afterwards published in the Transactions, I alluded to the curious fact, that a very large proportion, at least one in four, of the gouty patients who have come under my care to University College Hospital, had, at some period of their lives been affected with lead poisoning, and for the most part, followed the occupation of plumbers and painters (p. 282).

Garrod relinquished his claim in the third edition of his book, published in 1876. The retrospective credit he gave to Musgrave and Huxham was probably undeserved since these students of the Devonshire colic, while recognizing the association of the Devonshire colic with gout, did not know that lead was the cause. His belated but generous recognition of the contributions of Parry and Todd, was, unfortunately, offset by his failure to cite earlier writings on saturnine gout (291).

While acknowledging that lead was a cause of gout, even so independent a thinker as Garrod could not relinquish the traditional specter of alcohol. "Can lead impregnation induce gout without the cooperative aid of other predisposing causes, and more especially the use of fermented or alcoholic liquors?" he asked. "One of the most common exciting causes of an attack of gout is the drinking of an unusually large amount of an alcoholic fluid," was his rather ambiguous answer in 1859. In 1876 he was no longer prepared to answer the rhetorical question (291).

After Sydenham, the most distinguished English physican was William Heberden, George Baker's teacher at Cambridge (494). Writing of the colic of Poitou at the end of the eighteenth century, he seemed suspicious of Portuguese wines (364).

> For all my experience tends to make me believe with the learned and judicious Sir George Baker, that lead is the sole cause of this

distemper, though it be difficult in many cases to trace its admission into the stomach. Some of the worst fits of the colic, from which I ever saw the patient recover, when the cause was known, and could be avoided, have, by keeping out of its reach, never returned in many years; from which it is probable there was no fomes morbi left. I have likewise observed this happen in a more chronical kind of this colic, ere the limbs were become semiparalytic; the weakness of which gradually abated, and the pains never returned, after leaving off the use of white Lisbon wine, the drinking of a pint of which every day was conjectured to have brought on this malady (pp. 75–76).

From this passage and a similar statement under the heading "Colica Pictonum," it is evident that William Heberden, like Ferdinando Warner and George Baker, suspected the Portuguese wines of being particularly prone to producing the colic. Heberden also condemned these wines as a cause of gout, but did not consider lead a possible common cause of both gout and colic. In accord with his times, Herberden understood gout to be a diathesis involving many organ systems other than the joints. He summarized irregular gout as follows:

The cramp may also be reckoned one of the certain attendants upon the gout. Flatulencies, heart burn, indigestion, loss of appetite, sickness, vomiting, acidities, with pains of the stomach and bowels, giddiness, confusion and noises in the head, numbness of the limbs, epilepsies, palsies, apoplexies, inquietude, universal aches, wasting of the flesh and strength, and lowness of the spirits, are symptoms, some of which often attend the fit, and some follow it; and most of them are the lot of old gouty patients, who have moreover the prospect of entailing all these upon their posterity (pp. 35–36).

Heberden did not discern the saturnine component in his own description. Nevertheless, as with the colic, he suspected Portuguese wine as the cause of irregular gout.

The logic of the times was sometimes remarkably convoluted. If a particular wine was likely to produce articular gout, whether one recommended that wine or not would depend on whether the gouty paroxysm was more dangerous than its suppression. By such reasoning Spilsbury condemned the use of Madeira as a halfway measure. Since the wine would only draw gout out of the stomach into the foot, he opposed its use. Spilsbury advocated treating gout of the stomach with his antimony-mercury drops to nip the malefactor in the bud. He developed his argument as follows (702):

> The uncertainty relative to the humor of the gout is also apparent in the very mode of their proceedings to force the enemy from his residence, otherwise Madeira wine never would be indiscriminantly recommended; . . . why drive it out of the stomach, only to lodge it in another part of the body? why not attempt to stifle the hydra in its infancy, and prevent his growth; at least endeavor to weaken him in his first workings, when the stomach sounds the alarm at the enemy's approach? Not a fly, when he quavers on the cobweb, gives surer notice to the spider that his prey is nigh, than the sickness, and uneasy sensation, felt in the stomach, indicates that a something is breeding which nature is terrified at, and would, if possible, shun (p. 45).

By intricate reasoning this "chymist" acknowledged that colic preceded the gout and that articular gout was a consequence particularly of Madeira wine. He too, however, was not prepared to implicate adulterants in the imported beverage. This pharmaceutical entrepreneur showed even bolder, if somewhat contradictory, insights later in his treatise when he asserted:

> It is obvious Gout in the Feet is a distinct disorder from that generally complained of in the stomach; and although time immemorial has sanctified a farce commonly acted, of expelling the gouty humor out of the stomach down into the feet, . . . yet I will be bold to say, a fit of the Gout in the Feet cannot be produced by the medical arts used to draw it out of the stomach, without they first can explain what the hocus pocus matter is composed of (p. 87).

Such iconoclastic thinking by a paraprofessional did not merit a direct response from the medical profession, but a century later "gout of the stomach" was quietly deleted from the medical lexicon.

Dr. Oliver of Bath also took up the cudgel against port. Employing an early form of aversion therapy, he saw to it that his gout patients reduced their consumption. William Grant quotes Oliver on the use of emetics (325): "'In order,' says he, 'to work off the vomit with port wine and water, by which I obtain two advantages: first a discharge of the turbid matter, and then I often give my patients an aversion to port wine for some time afterwards'" (p. 31).

The attack on Portuguese wines intensified during the nineteenth century. Lead shot continued to be found in wine bottled in Madeira as late as 1819 (1). In 1841, students at the University of Pennsylvania were taught that not gluttony nor venery but affection for port brought the gout on Britain's leading citizens (124). Garrod summarized his views on alcoholic beverages as follows (291):

> My own experience of the relative power of alcoholic liquors in inducing gout amounts to this, that the wines ordinarily drunk in this country, as port, sherry, and other stronger varieties, are the most potent in their operation. . . . A few years liberal indulgence in port wine will often produce gout, where no trace can be discovered in any family branch. . . . Cider and similar beverages will also act to some extent as predisposing causes of gout and I am informed that in Devonshire the malady is by no means infrequent (pp. 265–67).

The lessons of George Baker concerning the Devonshire colic had been learned well enough to control the colic but not sufficiently to prevent saturnine gout. Accusations mounted against imports from Portugal. In his *Meditations on Gout* published in 1897 George H. Ellwanger wrote (226):

> What renders Port especially harmful, apart from the natural richness of the wine itself, is the adventitious alcohol it always contains, with frequently extraneous sugar and other foreign ingredients. . . . The undue proportion of Gout that has long existed in England as compared with other countries, can be traced largely to the revolution of 1688 and this addition of extraneous spirit; previous to which, and up to the date of the Methuen Treaty, the "claret" of France had been the general beverage among the wine-drinkers of Great Britain. Since 1688 the duty on French wines was raised from 1s.4d. to 4s.10d. per gallon, or three hundred and sixty percent; and by the Methuen Treaty of 1703, the gates were opened wide by gouty Queen Anne for Port and its boon companion,—the produce of Portugal being received at a rate of one third less than that of France. . . .
> . . . From 1787 to 1810, the largest amount of port was drunk in Great Britain; the greatest quantity ever exported from Portugal was in 1825, when 40,277 tuns, equivalent to forty thousand cases of Gout, were shipped to England (pp. 134–37).

This English journalist (658) thus recognized that the Treaty of Methuen was responsible for the influx of Portuguese wines into England. In exchange for eased regulations on the importation of English wool into Portugal, the duties on Portuguese wine were preferentially reduced. Port soon became the choice of the English gentry. Between 1704 and 1785, 65 percent of the wine consumed in England was Portugese while only 4 percent was French (704). Ellwanger further noted that the Portuguese were not subject to the gout although they consumed their own port in appreciable quantities. He attributed the difference in foreign and domestic sequelae to the adulteration of wine for export. "The excuse made for thus vitiating the wine," he explained, "is that it renders it better able to withstand the fatigue of the voyage" (p. 137).

Ellwanger did not know that lead was the traditional and most effective stabilizing additive for Portuguese export wines but was aware of the possibility.

> A third and frequent factor is lead poisoning, it having been observed that type-setters, plumbers, house painters, and workers in lead-mills are particularly subject to the disease. This is often more the case in England than in foreign countries, and in London still more than in other cities of the Kingdom, which leads to the belief that the operation of certain gout producing causes, less frequent elsewhere, is largely assisted by it (pp. 15–16).

The possibility that lead was the contaminant in Portuguese wine was tested by Gene Ball in 1971. In several samples of aged Port wines preserved for English connoisseurs, Ball found extraordinary quantities of lead. An explanation for the English epidemic of gout was at hand (39). It seems likely that more Englishmen sustained excessive exposure to lead than even Garrod suspected. Irregular gout might well have been saturnine. Vast quantities of lead had been consumed by the English for centuries in the normal exercise of their well known talent for luxurious living.

The etiologic role of lead in gout was, however, never as firmly established as it was for colic followed by palsy. Gout remained a nebulous entity, but as medicine advanced, nonarticular gout largely fell by the wayside. Only renal disease remained to torment the patient and baffle the doctors. Of little concern to prescientific physicians who considered this secretory organ no different from other glands, the kidney, too, was ensconced in centuries of misconception and ambiguity. Alcohol stood condemned for causing kidney disease as well as gout and colic. The sorting out of etiologic factors in kidney disease is still incomplete. The role of lead consequently remains the source of continuing controversy. In order to understand the nature of contemporary debates, it is helpful to review the history of medical concepts of the urinary secretion.

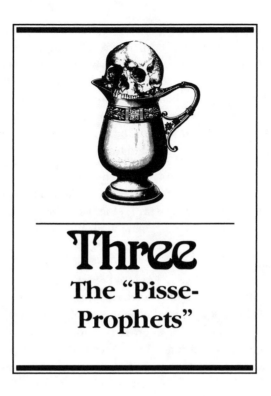

Three
The "Pisse-Prophets"

Lead Nephropathy

The Ancients described clinical consequences of lead responsible for dramatic symptoms. Recognition of more subtle effects had to await the application of chemistry to medicine and the development of pathologic anatomy in the nineteenth century. While "nephritis" did not mean the same thing in the seventeenth century that it does today, the first reference to nephritis as a possible consequence of lead was cited (with skepticism) by George Baker. Johann Jakob Wepfer (799) in 1671 wrote (33):

> Patients, . . . labouring under a bilious colic, which is apt to end in palsy, give me great trouble; but this happens abroad, rather than at home. . . . There are likewise in those parts a greater number of gouty and nephritic patients; people of both sexes are more liable to convulsions. There is a monastery near us, where the fathers drink no other than white wine. Scarce one of them escapes the at-

tacks of this colic. Not long ago several dominican friars were affected by this disease, after drinking the wine of Alsace; and convulsions coming on, they were all killed by it. I have suspected the cause to have been the taenia sulphurata dulcis, that is, bismuth mixed with sulphur applied to the fumigation of wine. The same cause had formerly been suspected by Thomas Jordanus, as the source of this disease in Moravia; on account of a supposed similitude in the effects of bismuth, and lead (pp. 339–41).

To Wepfer "nephritis" undoubtedly meant urinary tract obstruction due to stones. Nevertheless, he must be credited with linking colic, palsy, encephalitis, gout, and nephritis with lead in wine. Wepfer appears to have been the first to make all those connections but his report excited little interest.

An association between kidney "sclerosis" and dropsy had been made by physicians from the time of Rufus of Ephesus in A.D. 200 (506). In the thirteenth century William of Saliceto recorded that (474): "The signs of induration of the kidneys are a lessening of the quantity of urine and a heaviness of the kidneys with a certain pain in the back. After a time the abdomen begins to be distended and later becomes dropsical" (p. 21). Even in ancient times, the protuberant abdomen in ascites or anasarca was relieved of its burden by tapping (paracentesis). The fine art of bloodletting was, by chance, sometimes practiced in conditions which would benefit from phlebotomy, that is, in heart failure or kidney disease with fluid retention (fig. 39).

The diagnostic value of the urine proved elusive, however, until 1827 when Richard Bright drew attention to protein (proteinuria) and blood (hematuria) in the urine, fixed specific gravity and, in 1836, elevation of the blood urea concentration (azotemia) as the sine qua non of renal disease (92, 93). He identified the characteristic features of chronic glomerulonephritis, which subsequently became known as "Bright's disease," and he made it possible to distinguish renal disease from other causes of dropsy, particularly heart failure and liver cirrhosis. In postmortem examinations Bright observed that gross structural abnormalities of the kidneys were associated with proteinuria. The microscope, invented two centuries earlier, was still not in general use for examination of pathologic tissues. Although patients dying after brief illnesses often had large, swollen kidneys, in chronic cases, the kidneys were small and "granular" in appearance (fig. 40). This typical end-stage kidney caused some confusion in cases of interstitial nephritis in which proteinuria was

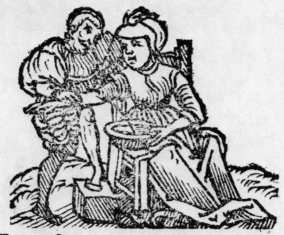

DE PHLEBOTOMIA, ET PRI-
mò de ætate fecandæ uenæ.
CAPVT XCV.

DEnus feptenus uix phlebotomum
petit annus,
Spiritus uberiorꝗ exit per phlebotomi-
am.   Spiri-

39. *Bleeding was standard therapy for nearly all diseases but may have proven effective in fluid retention due to heart or renal failure. From a 1551 edition of health hints from the* School of Salerno *(174).*

a late event but the gross appearance of the kidney at postmortem was the same. Because of the similarity of end-stage kidneys, glomerulone-phritis and interstitial nephritis were not easily distinguished at autopsy even with the benefit of microscopy.

Bright's derivation of pathophysiologic information from urinalysis shattered the venerable tradition of uroscopy or watercasting—divination by visual inspection of urine. Prognostication by inspection of urine can be traced to early Greek medicine. Hippocrates noted that "When bubbles settle on the surface of the urine, they indicate disease of the kidneys

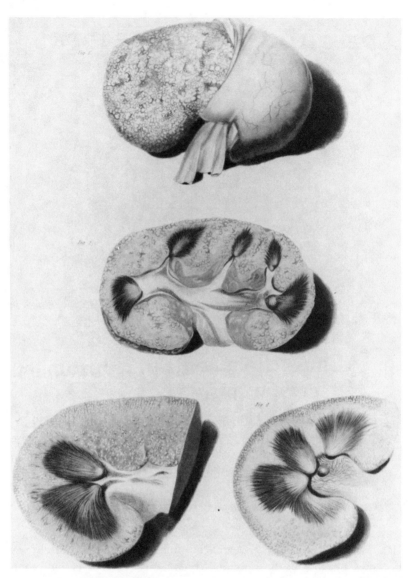

40. *The upper two kidneys, illustrated by Richard Bright in* Reports of Medical Cases, *published in 1827, were "granular," while the lower two showed an "opake, flaky deposit," presumably uric or oxalic acid. This gross pathology was later associated with interstitial nephritis. From the collection of the National Library of Medicine.*

DE ADMINISTRATIONE
Medicinæ. CAP. LVI.

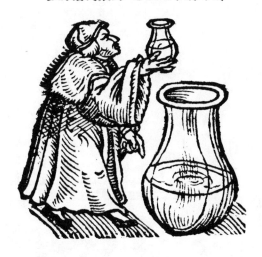

41. Gazing at a uroscopy flask identified the prescientific doctor as surely as the stethoscope identifies the modern physician. From a 1551 edition of health hints from the School of Salerno *(174).*

and the complaint will be protracted" (4). In 1849, the country surgeon and Latin scholar Francis Adams interpreted this passage as unequivocal evidence that the sage of Cos had recognized albuminuria. The conservative deductions of Hippocrates did not, however, limit the imaginations of later watercasters. "By the inspection of our urine," wrote Pliny in the first century after Christ, "we are able to give judgement and pronounce of health and disease" (607, p. 306). Gazing at a flask containing the urinary excretion was the hallmark of prescientific physicians (fig. 41). In one thirteenth-century watercolor the tumbling inverted uroscopy flask seems to carry the prognostic message "thumbs down" (fig. 42).

Uroscopy related to urinalysis as astrology did to astronomy. Ancient alchemical and humoral theories found expression in early studies of urine. The urinary excretion was subjected to the traditional spagyric techniques for analysis of matter—incineration and distillation. In the fifteenth century, Nicolas Cusanas advocated estimation of the specific gravity by weighing known volumes of urine (580). His mystical inter-

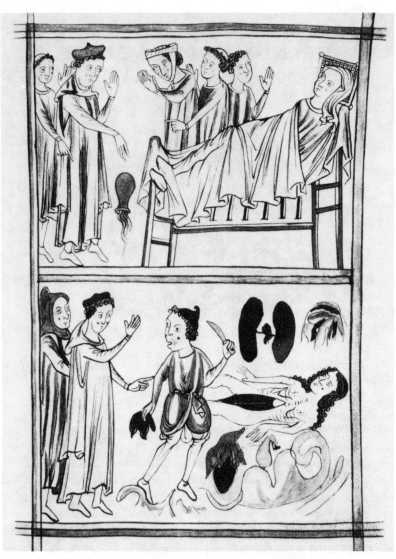

42. A tumbling uroscopy flask bodes ill for a medieval patient (above). *The kidneys are prominently displayed in an early anatomy lesson* (below). *Original in the Bodleian Library, about 1250 (380).*

pretations were, however, superseded by humoral analogies. The distillate of urine was considered to reflect the separate functions and diseases of the human body. Adepts could discern "spagyrical and anatomical man hidden in his own urine" (580). The uroscopy flask not only revealed the essence of the man, but the "Magus" saw the man as a distilling flask (fig. 43).

Even in the sixteenth century, progressive physicians chastised these soothsayers. "The Chymicall Physician affirmeth that such judgement of urine is monstrous," complained Bostocke in 1585, "and that the right judgement is to bee had after due separation thereof be made by fire: so that he see the matter for ech disease" (81, p. 92). But public clamor for wizardry could not be quelled by professional bickering.

John Gadbury, "student in Astrology and Physick," described over eighty-six urinary sediment patterns from which health could be forecast (fig. 44). His cryptic aphorisms were sometimes opaque (277): "Overmuch use of Women by Lust causes a rheumish Urine by decaying natural heat," he claimed (p. 37). At other times a glimmer of medical enlightenment could be discerned. His description of the "Seven causes of great quantity of Urine" suggests diabetes mellitus. Gadbury was also concerned with the appearance of urine in edematous states. Reaching toward questions for the future he wrote, "Fat like flesh, and dregs in the bottom shadowing, signifieth the Dropsie of cold, but if like Whey above, and clear in the middle, and shadowing beneath, it signifies hot Dropsie" (p. 42).

The seasoned uroscopist could prognosticate without ever seeing the patient. Not content with such feats, the adept embellished his prophecies with astrology. The person who delivered the urine was closely questioned in order to ascertain the correct oracular signs. If, for example, the urine was brought by a friend "moved of pity," then "the Lord of the Ascendent is Lord of the Urine and the Fifth House and his Lord is Lord of the Liver &c." (p. 44). The urine determined the horoscope. Practicing his trade during the early years of the Royal Society of London, Gadbury counted among his visitors a number of London's great scientists including Robert Hooke, who thought him "mad" (243).

Uroscopists confronted a skeptical public. In *The Pisse-Prophet or Certaine Pisse-Pot Lectures* of 1637, Thomas Brian, M.P., exposed the fraud of these charlatans. He told how "pisse-bearers" were deceived and urged his readers not to select physicians by their watercasting skills (90). "How great danger they put their lives into," he warned, "that adventure to take Physicke prescribed by the sight of Urine only" (p. 34).

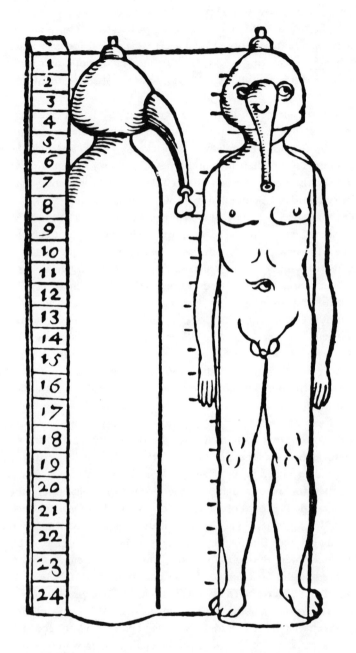

43. Man was the Anatomical Furnace *distilling urine in this Paracelsian tract on uroscopy of 1577 (583).*

Degrees of the URINE and URINAL.

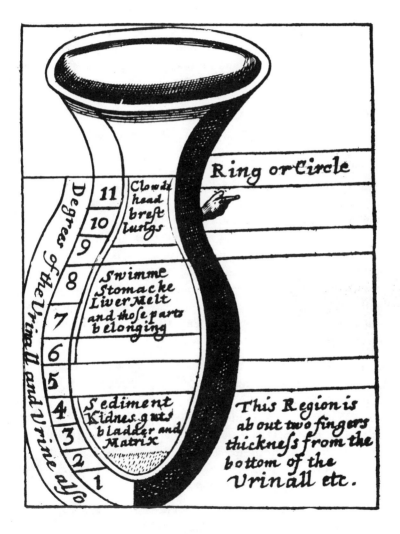

Ring or Circle

Degrees of the Urinall and Urine also

11 Clowds head breft lungs
10
9
8 Swimme Stomacke Liver Melt and those parts belonging
7
6
5
4 Sediment Kidnes g.ut.s bladder and Matrix
3
2
1

This Region is about two fingers thickness from the bottom of the Urinall etc.

44. *John Gadbury illustrated the fundamentals of watercasting in 1674 (277).*

But the awesome appeal of the uroscopist, as well as the thrifty avoidance of a house call, kept the demand for watercasting alive well into the eighteenth century.

The mystique of uroscopy sustained lofty public expectations. Meticulous, tedious observation was unequal to such showmanship. Fanciful interpretations of spurious data beguiled even the wisest of physicians. Boerhaave, for example, believed that "dropsical bodies attract water from the air" (722, p. 119), and he was convinced that gout was a cause of dropsy. Conjuring surrendered to science only with reluctance.

The appeal of the quick cure lost none of its luster even in the nineteenth century. Quack medicine fortunes could by won by mail-order uroscopy. Dr. Kilmer offered diagnosis by mail. From the appearance of the sediment, he prescribed his cure, a procedure which invariably confirmed his slogan, "Thousands have kidney trouble and don't know it!" (379). The "specific" for cloudy urine was Dr. Kilmer's Swamp-Root Kidney, Liver & Bladder Cure. Containing 12 percent alcohol, Swamp-Root was indeed "a diuretic to the kidneys." Its commercial advantage over the myriad of other cures hawked at the time may have come from the bas relief of a kidney emblazoned on the front of the bottle (fig. 45). Dr. Kilmer's nostrum not only stimulated sluggish kidneys but, after four decades, the national conscience. Swamp Root contributed to the call for the Federal Food and Drugs Act of 1906. Alcohol was harder for the body politic to stomach than was lead.

Richard Bright was not the first to detect protein in the urine. In 1673 Frederick Dekkers noted that clear urine sometimes formed a white coagulum when boiled with acetic acid (194). In 1725 Edward Strother reported a similar phenomenon (719):

> The Water of hysterick Women, and of Drunkards is easily distinguish'd, because the latter plac'd upon a Fire, or try'd with Alcalines, will not be precipitated: but the former will: From which Instance it appears, that altho' there is not Matter enough to send down a Sediment, yet there are some heterogeneous Particles contain'd in the Water of Hystericks; and, as Physicians are call'd forth to see all sorts of People, this may serve them as a Directory to distinguish between a Fit of Hystericks or Drunkenness (p. 403).

It would be presumptuous to regard this passage as the first report of the lack of proteinuria in the renal disease associated with alcohol. Such an interpretation would imply greater importance to the observation than Strother intended. It would be equally presumptuous to interpret

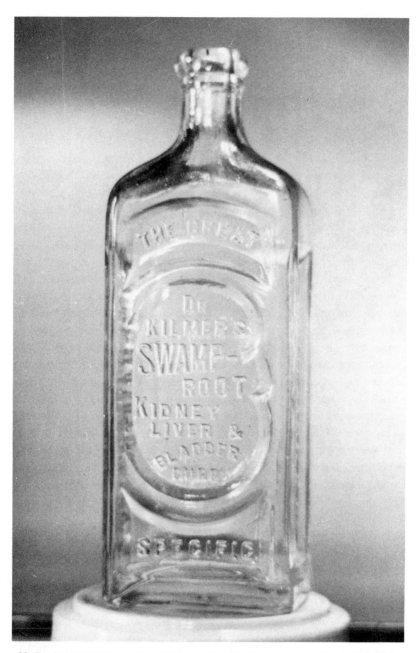

45. *Dr. Kilmer's Swamp-Root Kidney, Liver & Bladder Cure, about 1890. "The Great Specific" containing about 12 percent alcohol sustained enormous popularity until the Food and Drug Act of 1906. From the author's collection.*

Strother's "Hysterick" as a woman with lupus erythematosis or, perhaps, preeclampsia—both conditions associated with proteinuria and volatile behavior. In an intellectual environment of "received knowledge," observations not transmitted by the Ancients were considered at best trivial. In the tradition of uroscopy, the precipitate induced by fire was only of interest as another sediment from which fortunes might be told.

When word of heat-precipitable urine reached Boerhaave he had to verify the finding for himself. He boiled urine but could not confirm the rumor. Presumably he examined normal urine, free of protein, and his investigations therefore came to naught. The wrong question gave a spurious answer (418).

In 1764, a highly inquisitive Italian physician, Domenico Cotugno, noted again that heated urine formed a "coagulum" (161). His studies were an offshoot of investigations of cerebro-spinal fluid protein and he did not correlate the urinary abnormality with renal pathology (162).

Describing the case of a twenty-eight-year-old soldier who developed dropsy and oliguria five days after a fever, Cotugno concluded, "that all the fluids secreted from the blood in a human body, which are naturally not coagulable, are commonly rendered so by various causes, without being made turbid" (161, p. 32). Treatment with cream of tartar resulted in a prompt diuresis and recovery in his young patient. Cotugno attributed the recovery to the therapy, but today the patient's course would be considered a typical spontaneous remission of acute glomerulonephritis. In order to test his hypothesis that proteinuria was a non-specific finding, Cotugno examined the urine of diabetics. He was not disappointed. "Nor have I found this matter, which coagulates at the fire, in the encreased urine of dropsical persons alone," he reported. "But (though not in so considerable a degree) even in the urine of such as have been troubled with a Diabetes" (p. 36). Having tested the urine with heat (because he had previously observed the coagulable material in edema fluid), Cotugno concluded that urine and edema fluid were identical. Since his experiment met his predictions, he erroneously concluded that his hypothesis was correct.

In the absence of a meaningful context, the finding that urine sometimes coagulated led nowhere (265, 381). In 1798, William C. Cruikshank found that the urine of diabetics was often coagulated by either heat or nitric acid. In his extensive study of diabetes mellitus undertaken with John Rollo (652), Cruikshank observed that in diabetes with dropsy the urine "appeared to differ but little from the serum of the blood" (pp. 447–48). In dropsy associated with disease of the liver, on the other hand, the urine was not coagulable. But Cruikshank found no clinical insight in this critical observation.

More ambitious interpretations of urinary findings led to more profound misunderstandings. Where others feared to tread, Erasmus Darwin charged in. He publicized Cotugno's observations in England and correctly noted that proteinuria often precedes the dropsy (181). But his speculations on this subject were largely counterproductive. The circumstances under which Darwin first introduced his views were as unusual as the contributions themselves. In 1780 Erasmus published a manuscript of his recently deceased son, Charles, an uncle of the Charles Darwin of evolution theory fame. Two papers formed the body of this work—one the winner of the Gold Medal of the Aesculapian Society of Edinburgh and the other, Charles' dissertation. The posthumous publication was undertaken as a memorial to his son, whose untimely death followed a laceration received during participation in an anatomical dissection at the university. The father's efforts, however, failed to bring much honor to Charles.

Charles claimed that the kidneys played no part in the appearance of "saccharin" or heat-coagulable material in the urine. He believed that urine reached the bladder without entering the circulation or the kidney, a conclusion drawn after noting that the strange odor of urine after ingesting asparagus was carried to the bladder without being detectable in the blood. The urine of diabetics had the taste of sugar but their blood did not. Innocent of methodologic niceties, Charles concluded that there were direct nonvascular connections between the stomach and the bladder. He explained proteinuria by direct connections between edema fluid and the bladder. Both Darwins accepted the hypothesis that these channels were lymphatic vessels subject to retrograde flow; urine entered the bladder directly from the postulated vessels (180).

Erasmus did further mischief to posterity's view of his ill-fated son by attempting to wrest credit, for Charles, for the discovery of digitalis. He appended a detailed description of the use of foxglove to his son's manuscript, which was published five years before William Withering's historic treatise on the subject. In his account of digitalis, Withering did not overlook Darwin's ethical lapse (815). The misleading attribution was also noted by George Baker as soon as Withering's work was published in 1785 (36). The elder Darwin's experience with digitalis had been gained from consultations with Withering, a fellow member of the Lunar Society, whom he cordially detested (276, 815). Withering made no attempt to conceal his contempt for Darwin, venting his spleen with equal fury on Darwin's surviving son, Robert, whenever the opportunity presented (419). The frenetic animosity between Withering and the Darwins received more recognition than did Darwin's account of renal function. The elder Darwin's enduring vanity was unintentionally parodied in the epithet he insisted be engraved on his son's tomb: "Fame's boastful chissel, Fortune's silver plume,/ Mark but the mouldering urn, or deck the tomb:" (p. 135).

Erasmus Darwin was the last of the great gifted amateurs in science and Europe's most famous natural philosopher at the end of the eighteenth century (419). In alliance with Josiah Wedgewood he founded the Lunar Society dedicated to progress in science and industry. Notwithstanding the garbled venture into renal physiology, Darwin's visionary speculations more often proved right than wrong. He assisted James Watt in initiating the manufacture of steam engines and articulated a theory of evolution that was to be perfected by his grandson. Darwin's progressive attitudes toward human endeavor and human rights evoked a backlash from a public recoiling from the excesses of the French Revolution. His ideas were presented as didactic poetry, so turgid that succeeding generations of poets were inspired to create the Romantic Revolution (419). Shelley adopted Darwin's conception of the universe but rejected his versification. Darwin fell from the heights of adulation to become the butt of stinging satire. Subsequent generations of poets and philosophers have been reluctant to acknowledge their debt to such a progenitor.

With the Darwins, renal physiology regressed to Aristotelian conjecture. They ignored the observations of Marcello Malpighi, who had surmised functional significance from anatomic structure in 1669 (362). Malpighi injected the renal vasculature with black ink mixed with spirit of wine and described the glomeruli as "innumerable glands attached like apples to the blood vessels." He even noted the venules arising from tiny "globulis." But Malpighi could not make out the fine capillary loops within the "Malpighian bodies." Failing to appreciate the connections between glomeruli and tubules, he remained unclear as to exactly how urine was produced. He never doubted, however, that it was formed in the kidneys. In 1787 Murray Forbes asserted, "the urine is that solution separated by filtration in the kidnies" (263, p. 32). Lacking experimental evidence, Forbes' uncanny intuition was unpersuasive.

As long as authoritative opinion held that urine bypassed the kidneys en route to the bladder, it was difficult to attribute proteinuria to kidney disease (166). It remained for François Magendie to expose the myth of Darwin's imaginary lymphatic channels. Magendie pointed out that the failure to detect substances in blood that were found in urine was due to the insensitivity of the methods used. Material present in high concentrations in the urine, he observed, might be in very low concentration in the blood, requiring considerably more sensitivity for detection. Demonstrating once again that absence of evidence is not evidence of absence, Magendie rejected the hypothesis that undetectable retrograde lymphatic channels carry extracellular fluid and stomach contents directly to the bladder. He concluded that urine derived solely from the kidneys but he did not address the question of the origin of albuminous urine (497).

For most physicians proteinuria remained a curiosity which provoked few interesting questions (385, 445, 652) until the American-born William Charles Wells found coagulable urine in "the dropsy of scarlet fever." Having described a typical case of what today would be considered chronic glomerulonephritis, Wells rejected the renal hypothesis (798). "I have sometimes attributed such symptoms to an affliction of the kidnies, but perhaps improperly, as patients in this disease have, as frequently, severe pains in their limbs, particularly the lower" (p. 209). Confounded by the innumerable apparent causes of dropsy, Wells remained an optimist. "There is, indeed, an appearance here of a want of an entire uniformity in the operations of nature; but this appearance, in all probability, arises from a sufficiently long and accurate attention not having yet been given to the subject" (p. 216).

By 1813 Joseph Blackall recognized that the swelling of dropsy was not the result of a single disease and that a new classification was much needed (70).

> It has often occurred to me, that such an arrangement might be much facilitated, by a more accurate enquiry than has hitherto been made, into those remarkable properties of the urine, which characterize a large proportion of dropsies. Writers have spoken of the colour of that secretion, its quantity, its sediment; and it is a circumstance hardly credible that, amidst so much minute labour bestowed on these topics, the effect produced on it by the application of heat should have been so greatly overlooked. Yet the experiment is the easiest possible; and every practitioner may shortly convince

himself, beyond the possibility of doubt, that in a considerable number of dropsical cases the urine coagulates, like diluted serum of the blood (p. 4).

Blackall could not, however, decide whether the appearance of serum in urine was a defect of the blood or of the kidneys. "Whether the blood is presented for secretion in a vitiated state and in what manner vitiated, or the urinary organs themselves perform their office imperfectly, is at present not well ascertained" (p. 276). Blackall's chief contribution was not in providing the correct answer, but in framing the critical question. Once properly formulated the issue could be effectively examined.

The chemist William Prout was also aware that albumin in the urine was an abnormal finding associated with diabetes and dropsy (610). While urging routine urinalysis in medical patients, he, too, could not relate proteinuria to any specific disease. Prout noted the diminished urea and uric acid excretion in patients with renal disease, but he could not detect these compounds, or sugar, in the blood. He believed that diabetes was primarily a disease of the kidneys, an error attributable to both medical tradition and methodology.

The association of dropsy with proteinuria had a beneficial effect on the practice of medicine even before the renal origin was understood. Writing in the decades between Blackall and Bright, James Hamilton reported that dropsy accompanied by heat-coagulable urine was worsened by treatment with mercury. Particularly in the dropsy which followed scarlet fever he noted that mercury was often disastrous while phlebotomy and digitalis were effective in relieving dyspnea accompanying this type of fluid retention (350). By the process of trial and error Hamilton thus learned to avoid the nephrotoxic mercurial compounds in treating edema due to renal disease.

Hamilton did not believe that proteinuria signified kidney disease or that mercury acted directly on the kidneys. He envisioned both fluid retention and its mobilization as occurring at the site of sequestration. He was thus in no position to recognize that the detrimental effect of mercury in poststreptococcal dropsy was due to the superimposition of acute tubular necrosis on acute glomerulonephritis. Hamilton's empirical choices were nevertheless sound. Such views could not, however, gain wide support as long as his pathophysiology was intuitive.

Richard Bright avoided the dilemma created by an overabundance of anecdotes. He concentrated wholly on the pathologic anatomy of the kidneys in patients with dropsy and proteinuria, and he did not feel compelled to explain all forms of dropsy. By setting limited goals and bridling conjecture, Bright isolated the relationship between proteinuria and kidney damage. His research tool, the autopsy, became the cornerstone of nineteenth-century medical science. The narrow issue of renal disease revolutionized the whole of medical thinking; specialization became inevitable.

The reluctance of physicians to concede error was evident in the reception the profession gave Bright's monumental contribution. "The truth of the discovery has been obscured by doubts and hesitations, rather, than controverted by facts or arguments," observed Jonathan Osborne in 1834 (573, p. 12). Osborne not only made observations of his own in support of Bright's views, but noted that in cases of dropsy without coagulable urine the underlying disease was to be found in the liver or the heart. He further recognized that "acute nephritis," in the absence of proteinuria, was sometimes associated with "purulent deposit" or "suppurative inflammation of the kidney" (p. 16)—an early description of acute pyelonephritis. "The apathy with which the invaluable discoveries of Dr. Bright continue to be regarded by many is most unaccountable," lamented Robert Christison of Edinburgh, one of Bright's staunchest supporters (143). Christison felt it necessary to rebuke colleagues who continued to "call in question facts which have been long placed out of the reach of controversy" (p. iv). He recognized, too, the need to clearly differentiate between the symptom, dropsy, upon which Bright had focused attention, and the broader consequence of advanced kidney disease, uremia.

Despite initial resistance, the measurement of protein in urine became the universally accepted test for the presence of renal disease. But the limitations of the new methodology were soon apparent to Bright. By 1836 he recognized that not all renal diseases were associated with severe proteinuria (93). "I have certainly seen one or two cases," he noted, ". . . in which the condition of the kidney would have led me to expect albuminous urine, but in which it had not been found to exist" (p. 96).

The simplicity of the laboratory test for urinary protein was of such significance to clinical medicine that renal disease lacking proteinuria received little attention. Interstitial nephritis, such as that associated with lead or gout, does not induce proteinuria until the end stage is approached. The characteristic absence of proteinuria was not apparent in patients who came to the physician only as they were dying of uremia.

In Bright's extended studies of kidney disease as a cause of dropsy, he failed to examine the urine for protein in one case, that of a lead worker.

In Case 5 of his "Cases and Observations, Illustrative of Renal Disease Accompanied with the Secretion of Albuminous Urine," published in 1836, seizures and a "bilious disorder" (colic?) were prominent and dropsy was absent. The details of this case history are consistent with interstitial nephritis induced by lead rather than the glomerulonephritis typical of "Bright's disease." Case 5 is the one case in this remarkable series in which proteinuria might *not* be anticipated (93).

> Case 5. Death with convulsion and Coma—kidneys granulated. "Mr. P., an athletic young man of 25 years of age, by trade a plumber, came to Mr. Wheelwright, on the 6th of December last, complaining of dyspepsia, with some degree of dimness of sight. These symptoms being referred to biliary disorder, some aperient medicine, followed by bitter tonics was administered" (p. 110).

After death, apparently from uremia, Bright recorded abnormalities only in the kidneys which were:

> "rough and of a grey mottled appearance. This diseased structure was seen, on section, to extend throughout the substance of the organ: both kidneys were equally affected. The urine was, I regret to state, not particularly examined in this case; for there had not been the least tendency to dropsy during the progress of the disease, nor any complaint of pain in the loins to indicate its seat" (p. 111).

Bright deduced the pathophysiological significance of proteinuria without comprehending the nature of kidney function. In his day, the secretion of urine was considered to be the same as the secretion of any other gland. Even precise descriptions of the microscopic anatomy of the Malpighian body did not necessarily reveal functional significance. This insight was the contribution of William Bowman who, in 1842, reported that the nephron structure was ideally suited to filtration of the blood: the glomerular filtrate would flow down the tubule toward the bladder (86). And so the path was opened to analyzing the physiologic functions of this previously obscure organ.

For its importance to medicine, Bright's observations on the blood urea concentration were second only to his revelation of the significance of proteinuria. Robert Christison soon confirmed the value of measuring the blood urea as a laboratory indicator of renal failure (143). The test for urea became the mainstay of clinical diagnosis of renal failure. The major limitation of this test, now as much as in the nineteenth-century, is that elevations of the serum urea concentration do not occur until at least two-thirds of kidney function has been lost. In glomerulonephritis substantial proteinuria usually appears early in the course of the disease, sometimes accompanied by prominent fluid retention. In interstitial nephritis, on the other hand, proteinuria is usually minimal in quantity and frequently only manifest when the blood urea is elevated. The detection of nonglomerular disease before advanced renal failure is reached remains a clinical challenge.

Despite the rapid advances in understanding renal disease which followed Bright's work, kidney disease without proteinuria was largely ignored. Tubulointerstitial nephritis was recognized only by pathologists at postmortem examinations. Practitioners were preoccupied by the bewildering manifestations of the uremic syndrome, and laboratory diagnosis was restricted to urinalysis and the serum urea.

Tanquerel des Planches sparked a surge in clinical interest in plumbism with publication of his treatise on lead disease in 1838 (730). This encyclopedic review of 1,217 cases of lead poisoning remained the definitive work in the field for a century. Tanquerel was awarded the Montyon Prize for his contribution to occupational medicine and his book was promptly translated into English. Just as George Baker had brought acute lead colic to medical attention, Tanquerel publicized the delayed effects of lead. He pointed out that colic, arthralgia, paralysis, and encephalopathy are distinct entities which may appear independently in lead-poisoned individuals.

Tanquerel also described lead cachexia which was popularly mistaken for the emaciation due to tuberculosis and called "phthisic" (figs. 22–25). He noted the characteristic anemic pallor of plumbism which in English translation became "jaundice" and hence was confused with liver disease. Perhaps of most importance, Tanquerel described the slate-blue line on the gums often seen in lead workmen. With characteristic modesty, the English dubbed this sign "Burton's line" after Henry Burton who rediscovered the diagnostic finding two years after Tanquerel. Perhaps neither of these men merit full credit for the original description, since, in 1725, Edward Strother had recorded the presence of "black teeth . . . in House Painters [consequent to] the minerals so often swallowe'd down" (719, p. 431). Tanquerel countered John Bull with his own medical nationalism: he barely mentions George Baker in his otherwise comprehensive review of plumbism.

Physicians throughout the world began to search for sources of insidious lead poisoning. They were rewarded by the discovery that the sanitary amenities of the nineteenth century were not as hygienic as originally intended. Tanquerels's translator, Samuel L. Dana, found lead in the drinking water of Lowell, Massachusetts, and warned that the newly constructed aqueducts at Croton would bring similar troubles to New York City (730). Dana's prediction proved correct. By 1864, the Croton Aqueduct Department Engineers' Office endorsed Willard and Shaw's newly patented "tin lined lead pipe" (153). The problem in Lowell remained a point of contention for the Massachusetts Board of Health for half a century.

In England, James Bower Harrison published *Some Observations on the Contamination of Water by the Poison of Lead* in 1852 (358). Harrison's diligence unearthed lead pipes and cisterns where none had been suspected. The cumulative effect of contaminated drinking water was widely acknowledged but rarely corrected.

But as the reference point for all subsequent work in the field, Tanquerel's omissions proved as tenacious as his contributions; he never recognized saturnine gout or nephropathy. Tanquerel's description of lead "arthralgy" is considerably more ambiguous than his description of colic. However, there can be no doubt that he was not referring to gout. Using neither chemistry nor histology, Tanquerel, not surprisingly, failed to note the interstitial nephritis of lead. His important but flawed opus has proved difficult to correct.

In 1851, Robert Bentley Todd encountered a lead-poisoned patient with severe renal failure. He established the presence of uremia by extracting the serum from a blister created on the back of the neck. In the microscope, Todd saw urea crystals after reacting the alcohol extract of the serum with nitric acid. Lead poisoning was established by the lead line on the gums, a long history of colic, and symmetrical wrist drop (which he treated with Pemberton's arm splints [fig. 4]). But in accordance with contemporary thinking, Todd attributed the kidney disease to intemperance and exposure to cold. He was reluctant to assume that association meant causation, but this time causation was there. Todd did not suggest that all of the patient's symptoms might be attributed to lead (750).

The first description of lead-induced interstitial nephritis was published by Lancereaux in 1862 (436). Initially, Lancereaux reported a single case of lead poisoning in an artist who habitually held his paint brush in his mouth. After years of recurrent lead colic, the patient was overwhelmed by paralysis and encephalopathy. Apart from terminal albuminuria, renal disease was not evident during life, but at autopsy Lancereaux noted a remarkable atrophy of the renal cortex and tubular fibrosis. A year later, in a paper entitled "De l'alteration des reins dans l'intoxication saturnine," he described the interstitial nephritis in this patient in more detail along with three other cases of lead nephropathy (437). "The epithelium of the tubules are partly destroyed:" he observed, "the connective substance of the interstitium is very abundant (hypertrophied)."

In 1881 Lancereaux noted that "albuminuria is very frequent but not constant except in a certain phase of the renal alteration" (439). "Some of our patients," he continued, "presented with albumin in the urine only in the last days of their existence." The critical insight was that lead nephropathy is usually not associated with proteinuria (129–32, 446, 449, 468, 557, 570, 571, 595, 617, 635, 712) except under special circumstances—when uremia supervenes, or in the presence of heart failure or unrelated renal disease.

Transient proteinuria in association with lead colic had been noted as early as 1856. Typically, abdominal pain recurred for six to eight hours a day over a period of a month, each episode being accompanied by protein in the urine (56). Episodic proteinuria was also recognized with fever, encephalopathy, and a variety of acute stresses (56, 178, 585). But physicians who only saw patients during the acute attack were not necessarily aware of the transient nature of the urinary abnormality.

In 1863 Ollivier published a study entitled "De l'albuminurie saturnine," which failed to recognize the characteristic paucity of proteinuria in lead nephropathy. Ollivier considered lead-induced kidney disease simply another form of Bright's disease despite the absence of edema (567). In the wake of Lancereaux's report, he identified nine cases of proteinuria among thirty-seven patients with chronic lead intoxication.

Microscopic examination of the kidneys in Lancereaux's and Ollivier's cases was performed by Cornil who also collaborated with Charcot in studies of the gouty kidney (131). Although Cornil concluded that the "gouty kidney of Todd is nothing other than interstitial nephritis" (159, p. 35), he did not arrive at so clear a picture of lead nephropathy. In his thesis for admission to the Faculty of Medicine of the University of Paris (submitted simultaneously with Lancereaux's and Ollivier's theses in 1869), Cornil classified lead nephropathy as a "transient albuminuric nephritis" rather than as an interstitial nephritis. Lancereaux, alone, was left to defend the idea that lead nephropathy was distinct from the albuminuric forms of kidney disease.

Although Ollivier misconstrued proteinuria in lead nephropathy, he was the first to detect lead in the kidneys of experimental animals. He can be credited with the earliest description of experimental lead nephropathy but, at the same time, he merged proteinuria into the clinical description of the disease. This error was widely disseminated by German and French pathologists toward the end of the nineteenth century (298, 348, 460, 806). Proteinuria was catalogued along with the now-well-known symptoms of lead poisoning—colic, paralysis, encephalopathy, and gout (178, 449, 568). Few remembered that proteinuria was usually absent in plumbism (682).

The important distinction between lead nephropathy and Bright's disease was taught by the founder of neurology, Jean-Martin Charcot. In his earliest contributions to medical science, the eminent French physician focused his attention on saturnine gout and nephropathy. Working closely with Cornil, Charcot produced experimental lead nephropathy in animals and demonstrated that lead causes interstitial nephritis in guinea pigs in the absence of proteinuria (131). Charcot recognized the special group of kidney diseases which differed from the usual Bright's disease in that albuminuria, reduced urine production, and urinary casts were usually absent. He noted that interstitial nephritis was found in association with alcoholism, gout, and lead poisoning (127).

For a brief period Charcot's teaching prevailed on both sides of the Atlantic (712). But supported by Charcot's attribution of the discovery of lead nephropathy to Ollivier rather than to Lancereaux, the kidney disease induced by lead soon became associated with the more typical signs of Bright's disease.

In 1892 Lancereaux explained the confusion that resulted from Ollivier's work. Recalling his own 1862 report of interstitial nephritis in lead poisoning, he wrote, perhaps with undue modesty (440):

> Without in any way asserting the existence of any causal relationship between the two conditions, I, however, called the attention of the profession to the facts just stated. This led M. Ollivier to investigate the toxic action of lead in a series of experiments, the results of which were somewhat at variance with my own experience. He maintained that the administration of lead was followed by the appearance of albuminuria within a few weeks whilst I had been unable to detect the presence of albumen in the urine of any but very old standing cases of lead poisoning.

English physicians generally lost interest in saturnine nephropathy, although Thomas Oliver noted in his *Diseases of Occupation* of 1908, that proteinuria in plumbism occurs both transiently with colic and perma-

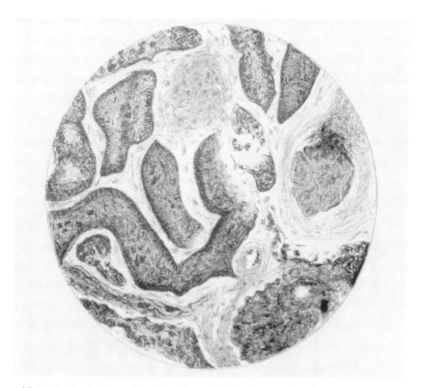

46. First illustration of lead nephropathy uncomplicated by gout, published by Thomas Oliver in 1908 (563).

nently as a sign of interstitial nephritis (563). Oliver was well aware that kidney disease was a major cause of death among English lead workers (A3) and published the first illustration of the histology of lead nephropathy uncomplicated by gout (fig. 46).

The last major monograph on lead to come out of the European experience of the nineteenth century was published by Legge and Goadby in 1912 (453). Colic, anemia, and muscle weakness were considered evidence of "mild" poisoning by these authors. Reviewing the mortality statistics for British lead workers for 1900 to 1902, Legge and Goadby noted that 7 percent of the deaths were ascribed to plumbism, 15 percent to circulatory diseases, and 11 percent to Bright's disease. Since only 2 percent of the deaths were "expected" from renal failure, Legge and Goadby concluded that Bright's disease was a common sequel of chronic lead exposure. Following World War I, as leadership in medicine shifted to the United States, this picture of industrial lead poisoning faded from view. Numerous reports of saturnine nephropathy, nevertheless, continued to appear in France (56, 178, 456, 504) and Germany (377, 480) during the great epoch of discovery of pathologic anatomy in Europe.

The forgetfulness of some English physicians was not entirely accidental. Dr. Alcock, "certifying factory surgeon for the district of Burslem," reported some method to the confusion about lead nephropathy (11). The correct diagnosis had the undesirable effect of requiring the insurance company to pay damage claims to the lead workers. Committed to the protection of the industry, Dr. Alcock went on to show how uncertain were the claims of lead nephropathy. The absence of proteinuria in the lead workers was, he asserted, ample evidence for the absence of renal disease. Advising employers how best to protect themselves from spurious claims, Dr. Alcock concluded, "A post-mortem examination will be valueless unless it happens to demonstrate the existence of independent organic lesions, discovery of which serves to exculpate the suspected lead." In the English-speaking countries, Bright's disease became synonymous with proteinuria. Fine distinctions were lost—except in Australia.

The Australian Experience

Lead nephropathy seemed largely of historical interest (22) until a curious epidemic of nephritis was recognized in young adults in Queensland, Australia. The first case of childhood lead poisoning had been observed near Brisbane in 1891 (301, 365). At the October 1897 meeting of the Medical Society of Queensland, three papers were presented describing children with severe neurologic manifestations of plumbism (328). In one case a postmortem examination had been obtained. The kidneys were small. "There was evidently present interstitial nephritis," Dr. Green reported, "and it is a matter of opinion as to the possibility of lead poisoning, which undoubtedly existed, being the causal factor."

Subsequently, an astonishingly high incidence of kidney disease was discovered among young adults in the rural areas around Brisbane (366–69). The renal failure was insidious, "Indeed so slight is the symptomatology in some cases," wrote Nye, "that medical men have failed to observe the writing on the wall because no albumin was found in the urine" (557). White frame Victorian houses were common in Australia at the time, but in Queensland, unlike other states, the houses were built on stilts for coolness and in order to control termite infestations (300, 328, 556, 754). The raised houses had closed verandas, ideal for confining

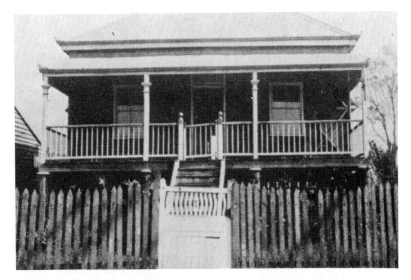

47. Australian children confined to the verandas of Queensland houses, as shown by J. L. Gibson in this 1908 illustration, succumbed to lead nephropathy as young adults (300).

small children while their mothers were busy in the house (fig. 47). Rainwater washing over the houses was sweetened by the dessicated paint and the children enjoyed tasting the rain dripping from the railings. Many of the victims had been nail biters as well and thus added another source of lead ingestion from the sunbaked white paint. The powdery paint brushed off easily, and by actual test 2 mg of lead could be measured on two fingers rubbed against the white railings (543). A history of lead poisoning in childhood was common among those who later developed kidney disease. Nye was convinced that the cause of the extraordinary incidence of interstitial nephritis among Queensland youth was lead ingested in childhood. Later epidemiologic studies, including analysis of bone for lead, confirmed these deductions (227–38, 365–69, 391).

Additional support for the etiologic role of lead in Queensland nephritis derived from use of the $CaNa_2EDTA$ (edetate) lead-mobilization test (227–31, 448). EDTA combines with lead in the body and the lead-chelate is excreted in the urine (609, 628, 629, 735). The ability of the one-day EDTA test to discriminate abnormal from normal body lead stores decreases as renal disease advances. However, by prolonging the urine collection to three days, diagnostic accuracy is possible even in advanced renal failure (238). Because more than 95 percent of the body lead is stored in the bones, it is likely that most of the mobilized lead derives from this reservoir (44, 227, 336, 373, 391, 663, 675, 694, 805, 808). On the other hand, the constant transfer of lead from bone to soft tissues may make the latter the more immediate source of chelated lead. Lead stored in the bones is continuously transferred through the blood to critical tissues such as the kidneys (803). This chronic endogenous exposure can induce organ damage many years after lead absorption has ceased and blood levels have fallen to acceptable limits. The EDTA test confirmed the presence of excessive body lead stores in Brisbane youth and provided a sensitive diagnostic test of particular value in the absence of overt symptoms of lead intoxication.

Half the Australian patients with lead nephropathy had gout, whereas gout is rare in patients with other forms of renal disease (227). "The gout was obviously not the cause of the renal disease," observed Henderson in 1958, "and its appearance in this series recalls the 'saturnine gout' of earlier writers" (368, p. 379). Emmerson too, noted that in contrast to ordinary gout, "Renal disease was invariable in lead gout and antedated the gouty arthritis" (229). Furthermore, the intrarenal microtophi, typical of the "gouty kidney," were found even in patients with lead nephropathy who had no history of gout (391).

The mass of evidence incriminating lead as the cause of the epidemic nephritis among Queensland youth was greeted by local officials with the same enthusiasm that had been accorded Baker's evidence concerning Devonshire colic. The Australian government's refusal to regulate the manufacture of lead paints led Nye to observe in 1933 (557):

> It is difficult to understand why no final conclusions were arrived at by the Federal investigators when a thorough and careful survey had been made over a period of two years, and when sufficient evidence had been collected to warrant a statement that lead poisoning from some source was a cause of chronic nephritis in Queensland. . . . It is well known that the lead industry is both powerful and important; but, although the proffered plea of financial stringency may be considered a very weak explanation for the cessation of the Federal investigation, it is hardly conceivable that mere policy or vested interests could influence the findings in such a vital question of public health (p. ix).

Nye found himself doubly frustrated; the government would neither accept the evidence of the lead etiology as conclusive, nor support the further investigation it deemed necessary—a dilemma not unknown in contemporary environmental controversies.

Nye's description of lead nephropathy in Queensland preceded by half a century the recognition of widespread lead poisoning among ghetto children in American cities. The children ingest paint chips from the crumbling walls of houses, a form of "pica"—the ingestion of non-nutritive materials such as clay, chalk, housepaint, and so forth. In 1981 alone, 22,000 children were found to have lead poisoning in the United States by blood lead surveillance programs (220). Renal disease is a minor manifestation of acute poisoning in childhood which is associated with catastrophic brain damage. These children show a loss in the urine of certain blood constituents that are normally retained by the kidney. Relatively sophisticated laboratory methods are required to demonstrate the renal dysfunction which includes aminoaciduria, glycosuria (112, 139, 141, 309, 491, 498, 611, 813), phosphaturia, and sometimes renal tubular acidosis. Such renal dysfunction is only seen when blood lead exceeds 150 μg/dl in children one to four years of age usually in the presence of severe cerebral symptoms of lead poisoning (545). Albuminuria is absent in the acute intoxication of childhood just as it is absent in the early phases of chronic nephropathy of adults. In adult lead nephropathy, such proximal tubule transport defects are far less prominent (164, 317, 382, 383, 793). The most important distinction between the childhood and adult forms of this disease is that within a few weeks of chelation therapy, in children, kidney function returns to normal. Reversal of renal damage is a slow and uncertain process in the more chronic lead nephropathy of adults.

To date, follow-up studies in the United States have failed to show any evidence of lasting kidney disease in young adults who exhibited lead poisoning in childhood. The significance of these negative findings is, however, doubtful. In one American follow-up study, objective evidence of lead exposure was lacking and reduced renal function was attributed to inadequate urine collections (740) while the other study was performed in children who had been deleaded by chelation therapy as soon as the diagnosis of lead poisoning had been established (553). Renal disease as a late complication of childhood lead poisoning has been seen in American children but has not been reported in the medical literature (J. Julian Chisolm, Jr., 1982, personal communication). The transition from acute lead nephropathy to chronic interstitial nephritis has also been demonstrated prospectively in experimental animals (26, 595).

The reason why Queensland children died of lead nephropathy as young adults while renal sequelae have not been reported in America remains unclear. Perhaps the Australian children had lower levels of Vitamin D, calcium, or iron in their diets, making them more vulnerable to the effects of lead. Even subtle deficiencies of these essential foodstuffs increase lead absorption (547). The mystery may be solved only when appropriate methods are used to find delayed renal disease in lead-poisoned children.

Pica is practiced not only among inner-city children, but throughout the world (35, 71). Recently, I encountered a forty-seven-year-old woman from East Orange, New Jersey, who had lead nephropathy, but whose source of lead resisted discovery (795). During a course of chelation therapy, it became apparent that lead exposure was continuing. She consistently denied occupational or household exposure and "moonshine" consumption. She did not own glazed ceramic kitchenware and her household water, by actual testing, contained very little lead. After a year of futile searching for the source of exposure, she was urged to bring in family members for examination. Rather than subject her family to medical examination, she confessed an unusual habit. While working in her backyard she habitually nibbled the garden soil. In winter, she ate continually from a paper bag filled with oven-dried soil. This soil contained high levels of lead, presumably coming from the paint in her adjacent frame house and from gasoline fumes in the urban environment. To the best of my knowledge this is the first description of geophagic lead nephropathy.

Lead nephropathy in adults has rarely been recognized in the United States outside of the Southern moonshine belt. In 1869 a case report by E. Paul Sale entitled "Albuminuria—saturnine poisoning" appeared in the *New Orleans Journal of Medicine* (665). Sale described renal disease associated with lead colic and proteinuria in a ship's painter. His brief but remarkable report demonstrated a knowledge of lead nephropathy not found again in the American medical literature for a hundred years. Sale's conclusions were based on William Roberts' *A Practical Treatise on Urinary and Renal Diseases*, published in Philadelphia in 1866. Roberts' work provided the most accurate review of lead and gout nephropathy available in the United States at the time (646). Sale not only realized that albuminuria was atypical of lead poisoning but was aware of the similarity of lead and gout nephropathy. He summarized his own experience with lead nephropathy (665):

> In examining the urine of the four cases of lead poisoning including the recent cases, and those of lead paralysis, which my wards contained, with a view to ascertain whether albumen was present,

it was discovered in Shawn's urine only, but in every one of these cases, the amount of renal secretion was in excess of the normal standard. These observations seem to support the opinions recently advanced in regard to the similarity of functional and structural change induced in the kidney by the gouty diathesis and the presence, or passage of lead in and through the system (pp. 727–28).

Despite the title of his paper, Sale appeared to have been aware that the absence of proteinuria in lead nephropathy differentiated it from Bright's disease, a subtlety which was often lost on succeeding generations of American physicians.

A single case of autopsy-proven interstitial nephritis due to occupational lead exposure was reported briefly in the *Transactions of the Pathological Society of Philadelphia* in 1877 (389). In 1895, lead nephropathy was believed to be the cause of death during an epidemic of acute lead poisoning arising from the use of chrome yellow (lead chromate) as a cake dye (711). At least sixteen patients were severely poisoned by one Philadelphia bakery. In one of the victims, lead was found in the kidneys but neither quantitative data nor histologic information was provided. A few other somewhat doubtful cases of lead nephropathy were cited toward the end of the nineteenth century (241, 490).

The dramatic acute manifestations of lead intoxication as well as the delay in appearance of interstitial nephritis conspired to keep renal disease due to lead in the background. While the acute transient renal failure associated with lead colic was sometimes noted, the slowly progressive interstitial nephritis in adults escaped further detection until the 1960s (534–40).

In industrial settings lead nephropathy has been recognized repeatedly among lead-poisoned adults in Europe (8–10, 38, 82, 283, 307, 335, 343, 454, 465, 468, 480, 589, 616–18, 634–38, 645, 657, 731, 766), often in association with gout and hypertension (454, 624, 634, 635), but until recently was virtually unknown in the United States (62, 91, 214, 330, 408, 443, 507, 521, 755, 819). In Europe, the kidney disease was usually identified because colic or gout brought medical attention to lead workers.

Prevailing opinion in the United States held that "industrial safeguards had made lead poisoning rare in adults even among lead workers" (221, p. 572). It was believed that lead nephropathy was not seen "because the prolonged and intense exposure to lead required to produce the associated disturbances would hardly be possible in industry in this country today" (214, p. 722). The possibility of serious organ damage in the absence of overt symptoms was considered remote (22).

One consequence of the complacency in this country has been that until recently no kidney biopsies were available for examination. In order to obtain human tissue for microscopy, Dr. Robert Goyer, an expert on lead and the kidney, had to examine biopsies obtained from Scandinavia (165). These patients had sustained excessive lead exposure working in a naval shipyard where they burned red lead paint from ships in the process of cutting them up for scrap metal. Fine structural alterations in proximal tubules and interstitial nephritis were found, but the reputedly pathagnomonic intranuclear inclusions were seen only in biopsies from workers who had been exposed for less than one year.

The explosion of science in medicine of twentieth-century America bypassed industrial lead nephropathy. The oversight was not, however, either isolated or accidental. Occupational safety remains largely under the control of employers—their physicians are committed to keeping the cost of preventive medicine down. Unions acquiesce in leaving the workers' health up to management and fail to perceive that the inevitable conflict of interest undermines employee protection. Studies of industrial hazards remain a cottage industry, an eighteenth-century relic in the modern era. Union contracts and, in some states, workmen's compensation laws assure both sides that the status quo will not be breached; health in the workplace is tenuous without a lawyer.

Inadequate diagnostic criteria contributed to the lack of recognition of occupational lead nephropathy in the United States (22, 91, 576), and saturnine gout was soon forgotten in aging textbooks. "In the United States," wrote William Osler, "chronic lead poisoning is frequently associated with arterio-sclerosis and contracted kidneys, but lead gout is comparatively rare. Gouty deposits are however, to be found in the big toe joint and in the kidneys in cases of chronic plumbism" (574, p. 398).

Following this description, the American medical literature reflected an increasingly disparate perception from that in Europe. It was generally believed that lead nephropathy and saturnine gout were nonexistent outside of the moonshine belt. The leading Harvard authority on lead, Walter Aub, observed that, "Gout has not been considered a usual complication of lead poisoning. . . . It may therefore, be possible that lead intoxication and a gouty diathesis are associated, although we have not observed it" (22, p. 203).

Aub measured the lead concentration in fifteen samples of homemade liquor and wine. In thirteen he found more than 1 mg of lead per liter and in four he reported between 18 and 75 mg of lead per liter. If Aub's patients were actually drinking these poisonous potations their physicians may have had very little opportunity to see the more protracted effects of plumbism. A less renowned colleague, nevertheless, recorded that over 25 percent of 385 cases of lead poisoning seen at the Massachusetts General Hospital between 1900 and 1939 had definite evidence of kidney disease (123).

I have recently examined kidney tissue from a lead worker whose death was attributed to alcohol withdrawal. For years the patient's wife and family physician believed that his bizarre behavior was due to lead at least as much as to alcohol. When the patient was admitted to the hospital because of seizures, a consulting internist rejected the diagnosis of lead encephalopathy because the blood lead was well within the then-current federal guidelines (755). The patient died shortly after admission to the hospital. At the family physician's insistence, postmortem tissues were analyzed for lead and toxic levels were found. The kidneys showed the characteristic changes of untreated acute lead intoxication (318)— lead inclusions in the nuclei of proximal tubule cells. This case demonstrates graphically the danger of inappropriate diagnostic criteria in cases of chronic lead poisoning.

In the case of another alcoholic lead worker we treated for lead nephropathy, marked behavioral improvement as well as improvement in renal function occurred after six months of chelation therapy. Over the previous decade this man had undergone repeated psychiatric hospitalizations. After changing jobs and receiving long-term chelation therapy, his aberrant behavior disappeared permanently. Both the patient and his psychiatrist were convinced that his mental disorder had been corrected by deleading. The psychiatrist concluded in retrospect that this patient's mental illness was an organic brain syndrome due to lead. "Insanity" due to lead was described in American mental institutions in the nineteenth but not in the twentieth century (613). Unfortunately even a meticulous medical history taken by an unsuspecting physician will rarely lead to a correct diagnosis. Misdirected questions elicit misleading answers.

As long as overt symptoms and signs of lead intoxication (colic, anemia, palsy, encephalopathy, and lead line) are required to diagnose lead toxicity, the association of lead with gout is also easily overlooked. Transiently positive laboratory tests, such as the blood lead level, have further confused the diagnosis of chronic low-dose lead poisoning. Throughout the world, saturnine gout has usually been identified only in patients who give a history of occupational exposure. Other sources of exposure have not been discovered, perhaps because they have not been specifically sought. While alcohol has long been associated with gout, the unpredictability of gout in drinkers has been explained by the quality and type of beverage rather than its sporadic contamination with lead (206, 221, 289, 302, 421, 478, 576, 608, 664, 809). The disappearance of saturnine gout from the American scene in the first half of this century may well have been due to inappropriate diagnostic criteria rather than to elimination of lead poisoning (91). Studies of the etiology of gout in which the EDTA lead mobilization test has been omitted may have to be repeated.

The present dilemma in the United States is a reversal of that in Australia a generation ago. Noting the marked reduction in lead poisoning among lead workers in Australia, Nye pleaded for elimination of lead-based paints to protect the children (557). "Does it not seem remarkable," he mused, "that no attempt has been made to save our children from the effects of this compound of lead which has proved so hazardous to workers?" Prior to 1978, the United States Government had taken broad steps to protect urban children from pica, but had paid little attention to their parents. In an era in which enormous governmental resources were mobilized to prevent childhood pica, does it not seem remarkable that so little effort was made to protect their parents from lead poisoning?

The kidney may not be the only organ in which lead-induced damage has been overlooked because of medical preoccupation with ethanol. There are, for example, suggestions in the older medical literature that lead produces heart disease (160, 376, 394, 693). The few cases of apparent lead-induced myocarditis which have surfaced are plagued by the same uncertainties that frustrated recognition of lead nephropathy—the absence of specific diagnostic techniques (239, 528, 626, 680, 715). Direct cardiac effects of lead are confounded by potential secondary effects on the heart of neurologic damage and hypertension. In adults the possible etiologic role of lead in chronic myocardial disease is further obscured by alcohol-induced cardiomyopathy. Once again, alcohol proved a more attractive villain. There is a tendency to ignore multiple etiologic factors in the production of disease once one etiology has been convincingly demonstrated. Just as the discovery of beriberi heart disease preempted, for a time, studies of the influence of alcohol on the heart, so identification of alcoholic cardiomyopathy may have concealed the effect of lead on the myocardium. The effect of alcohol on the heart obviously provides no information on the effect of lead (218), yet investigation of lead cardiotoxicity has languished. The successful production of myocardial damage in experimental animals (239) should stimulate reexamination of these effects in man. The finding that blood leads are higher in alcoholic than in nonalcoholic cirrhotics suggests that lead may contribute to more of the tribulations that befall alcoholics than is generally realized (499).

In children, the more subtle consequences of lead on the nervous system have received considerable attention in recent years (140). Alarming signs of subclinical poisoning, including permanent psychosocial dysfunction and nerve-conduction defects, have been found when sufficiently sensitive and rigorous techniques have been used (547). It seems more and more likely that whole groups of adults may be brain-damaged as a result of environmental lead.

The debate on this matter becomes contentious, even vituperous, when the question of delayed behavioral effects is raised (513). One side, led by Needleman (547), finds that even low levels of lead absorption in children significantly reduce intelligence later in life. The opposition, headed by C. B. Ernhart, contends that so such effect occurs in the absence of overt cerebral symptoms (240). This epidemiologic dispute has profound economic implications, since low-level exposure in children derives largely from lead in gasoline, while high-level exposure is usually acquired from lead-based paint. The lead industries support Ernhart, undaunted by her retraction of data and precipitous conversion to the "no effect" position. If Needleman is correct, lead should be removed from all gasoline. If Ernhart is correct, the problem probably arises from crumbling house paint; the lead derived from gasoline fumes serves as a background upon which more serious intoxication takes place.

The conflict between economics and health is evident in the World Health Organization position paper of 1977. The WHO *Environmental Health Criteria* document on *Lead* states that a blood lead of 50 to 60 μg/dl is the level below which no effect can be detected (819), although 30 μg/dl was considered the upper acceptable limit by most authorities in the United States at the time. WHO designated hemoglobin synthesis defects induced by lead as "obscure," implying that damage to blood should not be considered "poisoning." Such indifference to the effects of lead in children seems destined to recede into history. "Acceptable" blood levels have been progressively reduced (65) and are likely to be set at 20 μg/dl within a few years (605). The social price for high octane is greater than the public is willing to pay. The industry, represented by the International Lead Zinc Research Organization (ILZRO), can retard the pace of change, but neither influence nor affluence can alter its direction. ILZRO supports the research of some of the most outspoken skeptics of lead toxicity, including Hammond, Lerner, Gonick, Chisolm, and Ernhart (239).

Moonshine

Even after George Baker, lead in alcoholic drinks remained a source of poisoning throughout the world. Toward the end of the eighteenth century, John Fothergill cited English winemaking as particularly pernicious (266).

> In Graham's art of making British wines, are the following choice receipts:
>
> 1. To soften green wine. Put in some vinegar, wherein litharge has been well steeped, and put a quart of it into a tierce, and this will mend it, in summer especially.
>
> 2. To hinder wine from turning sour. Put a pound of melted lead in fair water into your cask pretty warm, and stop it close (p. 40).

In addition to legitimizing these "curious secrets belonging to the Art and Mystery of Vintners," Graham advised his readers that wine made of cowslip flowers was particularly efficacious for the treatment of palsy, convulsions, and the gout (319).

In 1820 Fredrick Accum reported in *A Treatise on Adulterations of Food, and Culinary Poisons* that lead poisoning from alcoholic drinks remained pervasive (1).

> The most dangerous adulteration of wine is by some preparations of lead, which possess the property of stopping the progress of acescence of wine, and also of rendering white wines, when muddy, transparent. I have good reason to state that lead is certainly used for this purpose. . . . The merchant or dealer who practices this dangerous sophistication, adds the crime of murder to that of fraud, and deliberately scatters the seeds of disease and death among those consumers who contribute to his emolument (p. 82).

Accum's revelations jolted reformers to investigations, if not regulations. In 1855, the Analytical Sanitary Commission, organized by the medical journal *The Lancet*, reported its findings after four years of study of *Food and its Adulterations* (360). The commission examined forty-six household groceries and discovered abundant evidence of lead in tea, cayenne pepper, snuff and confectionery. Colored candies were the worst offenders, 75 percent of one hundred samples showing the presence of white lead carbonate, red lead oxide or yellow chromate of lead. Sugared almonds, Oval Comforts, Kiss-Me-Nows, Ginger Palates, and peppermint sticks were heavily laced with lead. Candy fruits, swans, hats, and dancers, and chickens carried insidious poisoning to England's children. And these deadly treats violated no law.

Accum was not inclined to understatement. "There is *Death* in the Pot," was emblazoned across the title page of his treatise, surrounded by snakes and a leering skull (fig. 48). His biblical citation communicated the message even to the illiterate. The temperance movement picked up the theme and a few decades later, a newly reformed George Cruikshank used "poison in the pot," to illustrate a temperance broadside (fig. 49).

While in France increasingly stringent laws were passed to protect consumers from the accidental introduction of lead into wine, as late as 1875, Taylor bemoaned the fact that plumbism still occurred from the "tin foil" used for covering wine bottle casks (734): "In England the rule is caveat emptor" (p. 418). The danger of wine converting lead into soluble salts has recently been confirmed by X-ray diffraction studies of the powdery white residue commonly found on the foil-wrapped corks of choice vintages (771). Such contamination is exempt from federal regulation in the United States.

In the United States, the home production of whiskey has been considered as inalienable as the right to bear arms—not infrequently with similarly mortal effects. The art of home distillation had been honed to perfection by the Irish under the impetus of whiskey taxes first imposed by the English in 1662. Tacit approval of ingenious efforts to distill spirits and avoid excise taxes migrated to America with the earliest British settlers. The "little pot" still, or poteen, of the old country was adapted to the copper kettle of the new frontier (416). This cherished tradition of illicit whiskey is fondly recalled in American folklore. In Bexar County, Texas, "The Copper Kettle" is, according to Joan Baez, "first in the moonshine hit parade" (27).

> My Daddy he made whiskey
> My Grandaddy did too
> We ain't paid no whiskey tax
> Since seventeen-ninety-two

Lurking behind the dedication to individual freedom, there was a growing suspicion that free enterprise might sometimes endanger public

A TREATISE

ON

ADULTERATIONS OF FOOD,

AND

Culinary Poisons,

EXHIBITING

THE FRAUDULENT SOPHISTICATIONS

OF

BREAD, BEER, WINE, SPIRITUOUS LIQUORS, TEA, COFFEE,

Cream, Confectionery, Vinegar, Mustard, Pepper, Cheese, Olive Oil, Pickles,

AND OTHER ARTICLES EMPLOYED IN DOMESTIC ECONOMY.

AND

Methods of Detecting them.

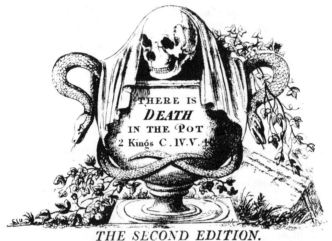

THE SECOND EDITION.

BY FREDRICK ACCUM,

Operative Chemist, Lecturer on Practical Chemistry, Mineralogy, and on Chemistry
applied to the Arts and Manufactures; Member of the Royal Irish Academy
Fellow of the Linnæan Society; Member of the Royal Academy of
Sciences, and of the Royal Society of Arts of Berlin, &c. &c.

London:

SOLD BY LONGMAN, HURST, REES, ORME, AND BROWN,

PATERNOSTER ROW.

1820.

48. Illustration from the title page of Fredrick Accum's 1820 Treatise on
Adulterations of Food, and Culinary Poisons . . . *(1)*

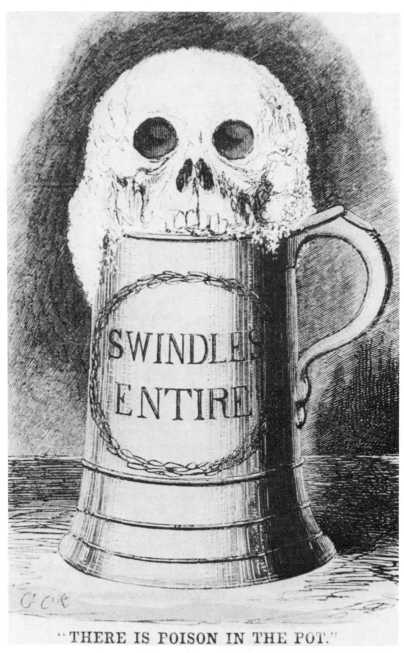

"THERE IS POISON IN THE POT."

49. Late in life, George Cruikshank became an ardent supporter of temperance. This broadside detail reiterates Accum's warning, "There is poison [sic] in the pot." The broadside lists lead among the adulterants of alcoholic brews that bring grief to the intemperate, about 1860. From the collection of the New York Public Library.

safety. The observations of Accum and Tanquerel were brought to popular attention in a modest monograph entitled, *Detection of Fraud and Protection of Health* by Dr. M. L. Byrn, published in 1852 (108). In this *Treatise on the Adulteration of Food and Drink*, Byrn detailed the sufferings of the unwary poisoned by lead used for food coloring. In normal times orange could be prepared from egg yolks. In times of scarcity, unscrupulous merchants resorted to red lead (562). Cheese, sugarplumbs, candies, and ice cream prepared by vendors were the chief offenders. Soda water, too, though a cooling draught on a hot summer day, might bring grief; its carbonic acid dissolved the lead pipes of the drugstore fountain. A Parisian epidemic of lead colic in the 1880s was attributed to seltzer (562). But Byrn's outrage at the plight of innocents poisoned in a sweetshop was mild compared to his horror at the perfidious adulteration of cider, brandy, and wine. He exhorted his readers to look to God and country for remedy from the treacherous practices of unprincipled wine merchants. Plagiarizing Fredrick Accum, Byrn exhorted his readers to righteous indignation.

> If to debase the current coin of the country be denounced as a criminal offense, what punishment should be awarded to those who convert into poison a liquid used for Holy Purposes, that which of all others is the most sacred thing on earth. Oh! will the day ever come when the God of nature will in vengeance look down on this wholesale murder? It seems that no law of man is made to prevent it (p. 70).

The United States government had more pressing concerns than to oversee occasional commercial excesses. Civil strife was threatening. The first liquor tax was passed in 1791 (416), but under the presidency of Thomas Jefferson the odious statute which had incited the whiskey Rebellion of 1794 was repealed.

Following the Civil War, Confederate army veterans could not always find legitimate enterprises to earn their livelihood. Some found it advantageous to exploit the persistent demand for illicit whiskey. The cottage industry in "white lightning" matured into a thriving business in contraband. An illustration from *Harper's Weekly* of December 7, 1867, shows Confederate army veterans at their stills in the backwoods of North Carolina (fig. 50).

With resolution of the First World War, the United States government expanded its protection of the moral fiber of its people and the proud tradition of southern corn whiskey grew to mythic proportions. Moon-

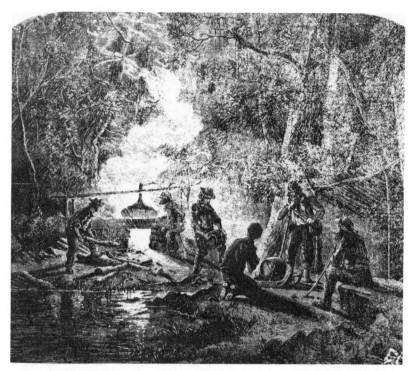

50. *Veterans of the Confederate army working a backwoods still in North Carolina as illustrated in an engraving after a sketch by A. W. Thompson in* Harper's Weekly, *December 7, 1867. "Moonshine" often contained massive amounts of lead leached from the soldered joints of the copper apparatus.*

shiners devoted to quality were forced into retirement in 1919 by Prohibition which made illegal whiskey enormously profitable. Quantity replaced quality and the heroic old-timer, the small operator, could only lament the poisonous mass-produced brews. Big business required modern methods. Truck radiators soon replaced hand-honed copper worms as condensers (762). Those familiar with the source of the new moonshine knew that lead poisoning would follow its warming glow. But as distribution reached beyond the neighborhood, the consumer, ignorant of the source, suffered the consequences.

Lead poisoning from contaminated wine prevalent over two millennia has not been entirely eliminated despite two centuries of publicity. Saturnism from alcoholic drinks continues to be a worldwide medical problem usually resulting from the accidental introduction of lead into homemade alcoholic beverages (66, 242, 417, 442, 591, 667). The acetic acid in wine leaches the lead from glazed containers that are reasonably safe for other liquids (3).

The danger of lead poisoning is not, however, limited to homemade or illicit brews. Lead glazes first appeared in Egypt in about 2000 B.C. and, soon thereafter, were widely used throughout Mesopotamia (554). Compounds of the metal proved a most versatile finish for pottery. A smooth, glossy surface was obtained after firing at low temperatures. Lead components were inexpensive and readily dissolved other coloring materials such as iron, copper, and antimony. But the stability of lead glazes depends on the techniques used in their preparation, as well as on the substances they contained. Medieval glazed pottery in Europe released massive quantities of lead into acidic solutions (322) while the gleaming ceramics so appealing to modern tourists in Italy, France, and Mexico not infrequently emanate lead along with glowing colors. Even fluids of weak acidity, such as coffee, can leach lead from export-ware glazed at low temperature (68). Using a standardized procedure (422), 25 percent of handcrafted earthenware and 10 percent of imported and commercial earthenware release hazardous quantities of lead (7100 ppm). While lead is almost universally used in ceramic glazes, the danger is largely confined to pottery fired at temperatures under 2200°F. The implications for health are unclear since neither the distribution of such pottery nor the frequency of its use with acid solutions is known.

Lead nephropathy in adults first received serious medical attention in the United States among moonshine whiskey consumers in the South. Anemia, colic, and seizures following consumption of illicitly distilled whiskey led to the initial diagnosis. Although Alice Hamilton had observed just after World War I that half of the lead cases at Johns Hopkins Hospital had gout (348), it was not until the 1960s that saturnine gout and nephropathy were examined in this country (40, 170, 347, 417, 423, 534–39). The blame ascribed to moonshine was devoid of the moralistic overtones that burdened victims of colic and the gout in the past. The moonshine consumers were clearly lead poisoned. Although the lead content of illicit whiskey is notoriously unpredictable (299), up to 74 mg of lead per liter has been found in southern "white lightning" (242). In the 1960s, most of the moonshiners admitted to southern Veterans Administration hospitals had both lead nephropathy and symptomatic gout (534–39, 822). Unlike the early gentlemanly Englishmen, the gouty Americans tended to come from the lower socioeconomic groups and were usually black (40). Hypertension was common and the gout began, on the average, twenty-four years sooner than in nonlead gouty patients.

Prior to these descriptions in the moonshine belt, it seems highly likely that lead encephalopathy was commonly interpreted as delerium tremens (170, 242), while lead colic was misdiagnosed as pancreatitis or alcoholic gastritis. The appendix (242, 563) or gall bladder (640, 793) was often removed when lead colic went unrecognized.

When the renal disease preceded the gout by many years, the effect of lead on the kidney was readily distinguished from that of uric acid. In more subtle cases lead poisoning was verified by EDTA testing (347). Morgan found that lead nephropathy could sometimes be reversed even in recalcitrant moonshine consumers by repeated therapeutic courses of EDTA (536). The Southern experience paralleled that in Australia. It showed that in adults lead nephropathy is a chronic and slowly progressive disease and that by using the EDTA lead-mobilization test, poisoning could be identified in the absence of overt lead intoxication.

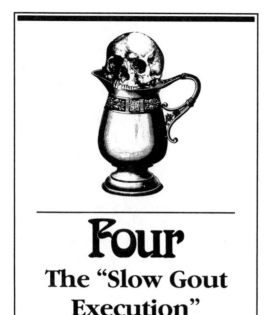

Four
The "Slow Gout Execution"

"The Morbific Matter"

Knowledge of gout is as old as history and controversy concerning its cause is as persistent as the disease. The gouty kidney was the first renal disease described in modern terms. Having identified the basic structural components of the nephron in 1669, Malpighi speculated on the mechanism of kidney damage in gout. He emphasized humoral factors (362).

> For the most part the abnormalities appearing in the urine spring from disease of the blood coming to the kidneys, and particularly those hereditary diseases whose diathesis is not developed in the structure of the kidney, but is in the blood. For a disease of this kind, as gout, frequently changes the kidney in accordance with the change of other parts (p. 261).

In 1675 a doctoral thesis by Buckingius reiterated this theme. Writing of "a man ailing from Arthritic Nephritis," Buckingius attributed the patient's kidney stone to wine (105). "Acidic particles of these wines, coming to the minute fibers of the glandular membrane and pores of the kidneys, depart hardened in the diverse manner according to the diversity of the matter" (p. 9). Finding a moral in this circumstance, Buckingius goes on to quote "the poet": "From loin-loosening Bacchus, and loin-loosening Venus, / is created loin-loosening Podagra" and "As Venus unmans the strength, / Thus abundance of wine debilitates the feet" (p. 10).

The spectacular visibility of gout was materially enhanced by Sydenham's pungent descriptions. Survivors had a surfeit of time to ponder the significance of the affliction. Tophi flaunted the presence of some "morbid matter." Striving to define this malevolent material, physicians began to formulate their views in chemical terms. Groping for a descriptive pathophysiology before chemistry had matured, one abstraction was heaped upon another, as if the choice of words could resolve questions that remained beyond formulation. Creative talent was expended in the reconciliation of fatuous theories. The more inclusive the argument the thinner the evidence.

The idea that gout resulted from some material within the body was ingrained in tradition. Seventeenth-century medical scholars strove to comprehend nature in terms set forth by Hippocrates and Galen, but the concept of humors barely hinted at the metabolic theories slowly being evolved. Natural phenomena had to be artfully molded to fit the ancient patterns of thought.

Struggling with Paracelsian concepts of causation, Hoffman attempted to make distinctions which could only be verified by chemistry not yet described (378).

> Acid wines which have abundant tartar, very greatly dispose to tartaric diseases, such as calculous, arthritis and gout (p. 46).
>
> If the serum abounds in particles adapted for silent and quiet contact and possessing many plane surfaces, they may easily grow together in the cold membranous parts (as, in the joints, kidneys, ureters or bladder) into a plaster-like stoney hardness. Thus arise the tophi in arthritis, and the calculi of the kidneys, urinary bladder and gall bladder (p. 64).

Such statements prodded chemists into developing meaningful answers. In 1743, Dale Ingram envisioned secretion of the "gouty matter" from joint membranes. He termed this tissue "membrana adiposa" and called the gouty matter a "coagulum" of the synovial secretion—a remarkable insight given available data (392):

These Saline Particles are chiefly produced from Debaucheries, unwholesome Air, Excess of Wine and spiritious Liquors, which causing a bad Digestion, Crudities, with sour Belchings &c. must necessarily arise; these being improv'd and nurse'd by Indolence, the Blood becomes impregnated with such Sort of Salts, as will at first cause an Obstruction in the Capsulae of the Membrana adiposa, with its Glands, and process of Time, break thro' them when mixing with the Oil they will cause a Coagulum (p. 41).

In several experiments Ingram reported that the addition of wine or vinegar (acetic acid) to joint "oil" induced the "coagulum." Had he used the word "precipitate" and described crystals, his fame would have been assured. The failure to follow through his ideas was a ticket to obscurity. Good ideas are commonplace; completed investigations rare.

Despite his superior insight, Ingram could not forego the almost obligatory attack on his predecessors.

I could wish that the Quackery which has almost crept into every Family, the Multitudes of Recipe's and Nostrums, the Grand-mother's worst Legacy, was less notorious in this Island. . . . Hence the immoderate Swelling of the Bills of Mortality; for (without Offence I hope) one might affirm that more Subjects are destroy'd by these Arcana in one Year, than have been kill'd in these last Four of War (p. 55).

A treatise on the gout not only enhanced its author's reputation but served as an effective form of advertising. The conventional tract included the author's secret cure. Ingram, a surgeon, selected phlebotomy and warm baths as the regimen of choice to which he added the surgical insertion of drains in the calf muscles in accordance with "the doctrine of issues."

By 1773 medical physiology was ripe for a concerted assault by the new breed of chemists. Rising above the foundations in alchemy, Boerhaave's protégé van Swieten articulated the challenge to science (722).

It will appear hereafter that there is something accumulated in the body, which derived afterwards to the feet, which produces the paraoxysms of the gout. . . . The particular nature of this cretaceous substance is disputed. Some imagine it to be a species of tartar as it seems similar to the caluculi in the bladder, which they imagine of a tartarous nature, as it seems to be increased by the free use of wines, in which tartar abounds (p. 137).

The chemical identification of uric acid in stones and urine by Carl Wilhelm Scheele in 1776 advanced rational analysis of the biochemistry of gout (672). The ancient idea of a "morbific matter" which was "thrown out" into the joints, received scientific support. But until uric acid was detected in the blood, speculation on the nature of the process ran rife. Murray Forbes attempted the chemical identification of uric acid in the blood in 1787 (263). "Upon mixing a few drachms of distilled vinegar with five or six ounces of serum, I have frequently observed, that after a day or two there were deposited some solid particles, which appeared in part to be the concreting acid; but the vescidity of the fluid is extremely unfavorable to the formation of crystals" (p. 32).

Having modified his test by acidification with muriatic acid (hydrochloric acid), Forbes was able to identify uric acid in urine with some regularity. But even this method was unreliable with blood. In a later edition of his work he retracted his earlier findings (264).

> It may be presumed that lithisiac [uric] acid is likewise in the circulation. To demonstrate the existence of it in the blood drawn from a vein, were, for several reasons, an undertaking of great difficulty. . . . When I formerly presumed to publish my sentiment upon this subject I thought I had been able to obtain concreting acid from serum, but now, after many varied attempts, I am not satisfied with my success (pp. 77–78).

In the absence of convincing evidence of a circulating substance, traditional concepts prevailed. Sir Charles Scudamore maintained that all the manifestations of irregular gout were part of a single disease. Despite his resistance to a chemical explanation of gout, Scudamore was moved by the monumental discoveries of the eighteenth century chemists to use biochemical methods in the analysis of disease. He also discerned renal disease in gout which appeared to be distinct from calculi and was characterized by "a remarkable deficiency of urea and uric acid" (676, p. 164) in the urine.

Over a decade before Richard Bright's classic description of renal disease, Sir Charles had connected gouty nephropathy with both proteinuria and urea retention. Despite uncertainty as to the origin of urinary protein, as early as 1816 Scudamore advised quantitative measurement of urinary protein excretion and determination of the specific gravity of the urine. Well ahead of his time, he stressed the value of twenty-four-hour urine collections. Failure to follow these suggestions led to confusion in clinical diagnosis for over a century. Scudamore's insights into the value of quantitative urinalysis proved far more durable than his concepts of gout. His approach anticipated Bright in providing the basis of modern renal pathophysiology. A final irony befell his contributions, however; his early linkage of proteinuria to the gouty kidney laid the foundation for persistent misunderstandings of the clinical presentation of interstitial nephritis (385, 581, 807). Despite meticulous and sophisticated studies, Scudamore added little to the practice of medicine.

Scudamore received not undeserved abuse for his failure to draw meaningful conclusions from his biochemical measurements. Unfortunately this paucity of insight led contemporaries to underestimate the value of biological chemistry. After attacking Scudamore personally, one contemporary critic proceeded with a global attack on the scientific approach to medicine (632).

> The legitimacy of any inference respecting the state of the blood, drawn from the examination of the urine, may be fairly denied. These remarks do not detract from the praise due the author [Scudamore], from his unwearied industry exhibited in the matter of the urine, but unfortunately, it has been a labour to no purpose, and the introduction of irrelevant details and illegitimate inferences from the state of the urine, has contributed much to mislead the author into the perplexity and misconception so conspicuous in his pathology, and also to swell out the volume, to the great annoyance and embarrassment of every reader (p. 52).

Not everyone was intimidated by the frustration and abuse Scudamore encountered. The challenge to understand the role of the kidneys remained. Richard Bright not only recognized that proteinuria arose from disease of the kidneys but further that in certain renal diseases protein in the urine was sparse. In 1836, he related the absence of proteinuria to disease involving uric acid. He noted that cases of renal disease without proteinuria were sometimes associated with urate precipitates in the urine (93).

Although Bright did not mention gout in these cases, his description of renal deposits at postmortem examination is consistent with later reports of "gouty kidney."

The kidney is sometimes simply contracted and hardened; sometimes loaded with an adventitious deposit; sometimes apparently degenerated throughout its whole texture; sometimes affected both with deposit, degeneration, and contraction. . . . I have certainly not always found the quantity of albumin increased in proportion to the apparent advance in the structural disease (p. 98).

The exceptions to proteinuria in Bright's disease, in the gifted physician's own view, included nephropathy in gout. The astuteness of Bright's observations seems all the more remarkable when it is remembered that his initial pathologic differentiation was made from gross dissections of postmortem kidneys.

The idea that gout arose from circulating uric acid remained appealing to many nineteenth-century physicians even though proof was beyond their chemical skills. To physicians steeped in the new science it seemed inescapable that a specific organic compound would be found in the blood which would explain the signs and symptoms of gout. Having identified the question, a sense of growing anticipation animated medical writing (587, 749). In 1842, Henry Bence-Jones stated the challenge that Garrod was to meet (60).

It seems likely that "when the question is fairly driven" chemistry will soon return an answer. But whether it be urea, uric acid or some previous substance out of which these are formed which exists in the blood, the quantity is so small and it is so quickly changed by the kidneys, that no satisfactory conclusion can be drawn from an examination of small quantities of blood.

Certainly in the gout, the one or other of these states must exist; either there is an excess of that substance which is capable of producing uric acid when it comes to the kidneys, which is passed during an attack of gout from the systemic capillaries to those of the kidneys, and there gives rise to the excess of uric acid which appears in the urine, or, which is more probable, urate of ammonia itself (formed from the metamorphosis of the tissues) exists in the blood in larger quantities than usual (p. 62).

The first clinically practical method for measuring uric acid in blood was developed by Garrod whose "uric acid thread experiment" revolutionized not only medical notions of gout but fundamental concepts of disease (286). Garrod standardized a procedure for detecting uric acid in serum. He used acetic instead of muriatic acid and added a piece of thread to the evaporating dish on which crystals could form. Though only crudely quantitative, this test permitted consistent detection of uric acid in concentrations of 9 mg/dl or higher (291). Not only could gout subsequently be correlated with the serum uric acid, but unrelated disease previously designated "irregular gout" could be separated from the gouty diathesis.

In 1848 Garrod emphasized the intimate relationship between gout and kidney disease. He noted that renal damage was frequently present in gout and that hyperuricemia was invariably present in kidney disease. Garrod did not, however, presume to deduce causation from association. But the distinction betwen Bright's disease and the gouty kidney did not escape his attention (285). "In gout, the blood sometimes contains a little urea," he noted, adding parenthetically, "no albumin being present in the urine" (p. 89)—renal failure without proteinuria.

After convincing himself, as Bright, Christison, and Rees had done before, that "a little urea" in the serum was abnormal, Garrod concluded that "urea may sometimes be retained in the system to a considerable extent, without existence of any such disease of the kidneys as is made known by the presence of albumin" (p. 96). Thus, Garrod recorded the physiologic concomitants of interstitial nephritis which distinguish the renal disease of gout from glomerulonephritis.

In his classic description of gout published in 1859, Garrod emphasized the fact that no less than one-quarter of his patients were lead workers who had, at one time or another, exhibited symptoms of plumbism (289). In 1870, he increased this estimate to one-third (290). The implications of this crucial observation, contradicting both George Baker and Tanquerel des Planches, never seems to have been fully appreciated.

Believing that lead played a more than casual role in the widespread gout of nineteenth-century England, Garrod examined the effect of orally administered lead acetate on the renal excretion of uric acid. At that time, the sugar of lead still had a prominent place in therapeutics. Garrod found that lead induces hyperuricemia by reducing renal urate excretion, thereby predisposing to attacks of gout. He also established the fact that gout patients tend to excrete less, rather than more, uric acid than do normal subjects.

In the 125 years since Garod made these observations, little new insight has been added to our knowledge of the effect of lead on uric acid. Intensive modern investigation of uric acid excretion in gout patients (without known lead intoxication) has established that at least 80 percent of such patients excrete less than the "normal" 600 mg of uric acid per day (80). The extent to which lead contributes to these findings is unknown. At least some of the overexcretors have been shown to have a genetically controlled enzyme defect which leads to excessive uric acid production (232, 233). Modern studies have usually confirmed the diminished uric acid excretion in lead nephropathy but sometimes have suggested that an increase in uric acid production also contributes to the hyperuricemia of lead intoxication (228, 236, 478, 480). An increase in metabolism of uric acid precursors, the building blocks of DNA and RNA, has been demonstrated to be induced by lead, at least in the test tube (239, 324). The full spectrum of molecular events which herald cellular damage from lead remain to be determined.

Although Garrod's contribution to understanding gout cannot be overestimated, hyperuricemia is neither necessary nor sufficient to define the disease. No sharp cutoff can be determined for serum uric acid levels to distinguish gouty individuals unequivocally from normal subjects. An elevated serum uric acid level is not unusual in the nongouty population (402). Moreover, less than a third of patients with acute gouty arthritis have distinct elevations of their serum uric acids. Five percent of men with elevated uric acid levels have evidence of renal disease but it is unclear whether this is higher than in the normouricemic population.

It has long been recognized that both genetic and environmental factors play a role in the etiology of gout. Familial gout is considered to be of genetic origin and is called "primary" (342). When gout appears sporadically or is elicited by identifiable causes of hyperuricemia such as blood disease or lead intoxication, it is considered to be "secondary." These concepts of primary and secondary gout are largely determined by the methods used to identify "secondary." But just as association does not prove causation, so the absence of identification of a cause does not prove the absence of the cause.

The factors identified as inciting gout depend very greatly on exactly what is looked for. The idea that gout is transmitted from father to son has been repeated since Hippocrates, but scientifically sound support for this belief has yet to be found. Despite universal repetition, compelling evidence that gout is inherited is still lacking. Differences in serum uric acid levels between ethnic groups are usually interpreted as genetically determined, although systematic environmental differences such as dietary habits have never been rigorously excluded. At best, available evidence suggests that gout results from environmental influences in susceptible individuals (74, 332).

The effects of lead on the serum uric acid level have been obscured by the finding that a variety of common foodstuffs also diminish uric acid excretion. Even in the absence of gout, hyperuricemia may be caused by the use of alcohol (257). It is clear that lead is not the only substance in alcoholic drinks which tends to increase uric acid in the blood. Ethanol itself transiently increases the serum uric acid concentration (454, 492). The mechanism appears to be indirect; ethanol increases the serum lactate level which in turn reduces the renal excretion of uric acid. Gluttony and fasting alike contribute to the acute hyperuricemia of alcohol excess (558). Hyperlipemia was perhaps more common in eighteenth-century English imbibers than in present day alcoholics who more commonly sustain starvation ketosis. The renal consequences of both of these alimentary aberrations, however, are the same—decreased excretion and increased serum levels of uric acid. It has even been suggested that reducing the oxygen supply to tissues increases uric acid production by depleting cells of their energy currency, purine nucleotides (818). According to this view, cardiovascular collapse of any cause may increase purine degradation and, thus, increase uric acid production. A variety of drugs including aspirin and diuretics also contribute to transient hyperuricemia (187). But the sustained hyperuricemia of chronic gout is at least sometimes more readily explained by the long-lasting effects of lead.

For centuries, wine was considered a major cause of gout but at present this association has all but vanished from the medical literature. The possibility remains that not wine but a sporadic contaminant of wine was the culprit. Lead is a likely candidate as the substance in wine which caused the gout. In concert with other factors which predispose to hyperuricemia and acute attacks, the contribution of lead may often be decisive. Inconstant adulteration of liquors with lead throughout history may be responsible for the inconsistent association of wine with gout.

If lead is a cause of the sporadic association of wine with gout, this contaminant could also account for the enormously varied symptomatology traditionally associated with gout. "Irregular," "retrocedent," and "atonic" gout refer to symptoms which can no longer be attributed to the "gouty diathesis."

The Gouty Kidney

Although "irregular gout" has vanished from the physician's vocabulary, the effect of uric acid on the kidney remains the subject of controversy. In the past, gout was not only believed to be a common cause of renal disease (292), but renal disease was also widely viewed as the major cause of death in gout (73, 96, 97, 425, 461, 496, 653, 673, 725, 727, 728, 821). Some physicians still believe that hyperuricemia per se leads to renal disease (152, 210, 305, 415, 426, 787, 796), while others contend that in the absence of kidney stones or intrarenal urate deposits, kidney impairment in gout is due to pyelonephritis, hypertension, or other concurrent disease (62, 255, 321, 415, 584, 656, 823–25). It has proven enormously difficult to distinguish causation from association. In 1979, Fessel summarized the conclusions of a long-term follow-up of patients with hyperuricemia conducted in California. "The widely held concept that azotemia is a long term outcome of hyperuricemia that is of usual degree, is unfounded on observation" (255, p. 79).

How can the conflicting perceptions of so ancient a disease be explained? Some of the controversy stemmed from the fact that at least three different mechanisms of renal damage operate in gout. When lodged in the ureter, uric acid stones produce the extreme pain of ureteral colic. As with intestinal colic and acute gout, such pain could hardly go unnoticed even in centuries past. The associating of ureteral colic with gout was familiar to Sydenham (592).

> Nor does the Pain, the lameness, and the obstructed motion of the affected parts, the Sickness and other Symptoms describ'd compleat the Tragedy of this Disease: For it breeds the Stone of the Kidnies in very many, either because the Sick long lies upon the Back, or because the Organs of Secretion have ceas'd to perform their due Functions, or for that the Stone is made of the same kind of Matter, but which is the cause I shall not determine: whatever is the origin of the Disease, the Sick has sometimes many sad Contemplations, to know whether the Stone or the Gout is most severe; and sometimes the Stone hindering the passage of Water into the Bladder through the Urinary Passages kills him, not awaiting any longer upon the Slow Gout Execution (p. 95).

The renal consequences of the displaced "peccant matter" were at least as ominous as the gastrointestinal symptoms. Writing "Of The Gout" not long after Sydenham, John Quincy noted that "Arthriticks have many Symptoms in common with Nephriticks, having frequently Interchange from one to another" (615, p. 407). But only the obstruction of the urinary outflow tracts was implied by these descriptions. The more subtle forms of gouty nephropathy escaped detection.

Other forms of renal disease in gout were considerably more difficult to define as long as the normal histology and physiology of the kidney were unknown. Pathophysiologic mechanisms were consequently the subject of speculation. To derive accurate inferences from the array of random observations then available took considerable luck, as well as a modicum of brilliance. Murray Forbes was preeminant amongst the successful theorists. Having surmised glomerular filtration and hyperuricemia well before techniques were available for their detection, in 1787 (263). Forbes proceeded to describe the distinctive features of the gouty kidney before pathologic data had been assembled. He attributed the earliest recognition of the gouty kidney to de Haen, another of Boerhaave's protégés (264).

> Red sand deposited from the urine in the very act of secretion has often been found in the tubuli uriniferi. A case is reported by de Haen where the whole substance of these glands were loaded with this matter, which in the particular instance of this patient, who was severely afflicted with arthritic affection, he considered as the matter of gout (p. 86).

Although a gouty death was sometimes attributed to failure of the kidneys (659), four decades later Forbes' observations had still not been confirmed.

Following Richard Bright's 1827 description of the significance of proteinuria, European physicians began to evaluate kidney disease with more attention to anatomic-physiologic correlations. In 1839–41, P. F. O. Rayer published the first comprehensive text on the pathologic anatomy of the kidney, including a fine color lithograph of the granular, shrunken kidney of *néphrite goutteuse* (fig. 51, [625]). He was aware that proteinuria was unusual in gout and that edema was rare. In a postmortem examination of a gout patient with lead colic, Rayer recorded that proteinuria decreased as lead colic abated, but he failed to recognize the relationship of gout to saturnism.

Rayer described small urate grains in the renal cortex which, like those of Murray Forbes, have been subsequently interpreted as being tiny intrarenal stones. In the tradition of Scudamore, he classified gout nephropathy under albuminuric nephritis. Because his cortical granules have been considered microcalculi rather than intrarenal precipitates, Rayer's observations have been all but forgotten. This harsh fate was reinforced by Rayer's most distinguished student, Jean-Martin Charcot. In 1853, in defense of his doctoral thesis, Charcot praised Rayer for his original description of "néphrite goutteuse" (125), but a decade later he credited R. B.

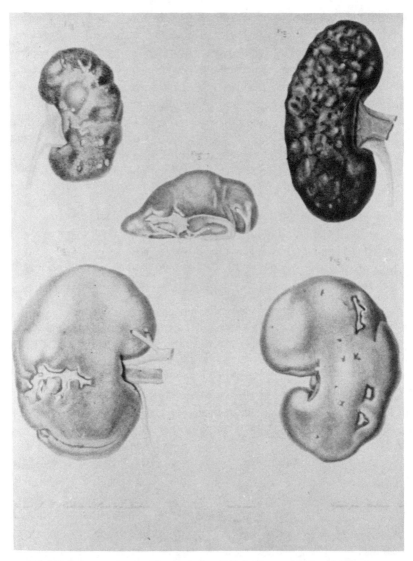

51. Néphrite goutteuse *illustrated by P. F. O. Rayer, 1839–41. The gross anatomy of the contracted, granular kidney in gout is consistent with advanced interstitial nephritis (625).*

Todd with coining the phrase "gouty kidney" (126). At the same time, Charcot attributed the first identification of intrarenal urate precipitates to his colleague Henri de Castelnau. The reason for the great French physician's lapse of generosity toward his old professor and mentor is nowhere evident.

In 1843, de Castelnau provided the first unequivocal description of the unique white striations in the gouty kidney which represented the uratic precipitates (121). He believed that this pathologic feature distinguished the gouty kidney from all other renal diseases. De Castelnau's description followed by 164 years Leeuwenhoek's visualization of crystals in tophi (484), by 46 years Wollaston's identification of the composition of the crystals (816), but preceded by 5 years Garrod's first measurements of uric acid in blood (285). In 1847, Todd rediscovered these urate deposits in the kidney to the wide acclaim of his English compatriots. In reality, Todd's contribution was not the discovery of the "gouty kidney," but his emphasis on the differences between the gouty kidney and Bright's disease (751). In a patient with heavy proteinuria Todd noted, "The existence of so large a quantity of albumen is quite exceptional in cases of gouty kidney" (p. 218). He attributed the proteinuria to severe rightsided heart failure—a conclusion consistent with modern interpretations.

In 1859, Garrod published anatomical illustrations of the shrunken end-stage kidney of gout (fig. 52). Apparently unaware at that time of de Haen's, Forbes', Rayer's and de Castelnau's earlier observations, Garrod claimed to have been the first to note the characteristic deposits in the gouty kidney in 1849 (289). Although he chemically identified urate in gouty kidneys, thereby proving de Castelnau's surmise, Garrod's published illustration did not show histologic detail; the uric acid streaks in the medulla were hardly discernible.

For Garrod, the gouty kidney and plumbism were allied conditions. At a meeting of the Pathological Society of London in 1856, he exhibited the gouty kidneys of a lead worker. The patient "was a painter by trade and was a great drunkard." His urine was initially free of albumin but "the tubuli were blocked up with urate of soda" (287, p. 97). Fourteen years later describing a case of saturnine gout, Garrod noted that lead produced a contracted kidney with little albuminuria (290).

Thus, he recognized that renal disease in gout was sometimes associated with lead, but he never emphasized the connection. Although responsible for contemporary awareness of saturnine gout, Garrod did not propose an etiologic role for lead in gout nephropathy. He recognized, however, that even slight proteinuria was unusual in gout, except transiently during the acute arthritic attack and late in the course of chronic gout (288).

In the second half of the nineteenth century, leadership in defining the pathology of gout shifted from England to France. In collaboration with

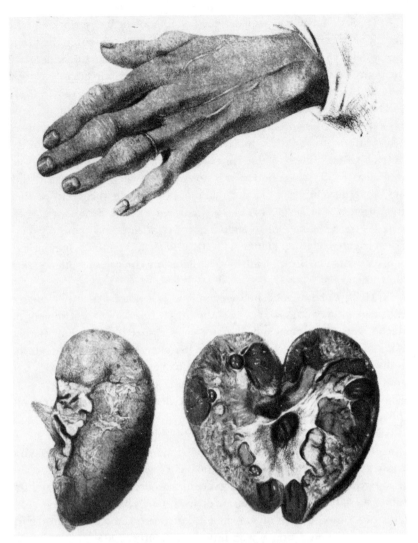

52. *Alfred Baring Garrod recognized kidney disease as a major cause of death in his gout patients, as shown in his 1859 lithographic illustration of granular kidneys (289).*

his intern at the Salpêtrière Hospital, André Victor Cornil, Charcot published the earliest (1864) illustrations of urate deposits in the gouty kidney as seen in the microscope (127). He noted that such deposits often appeared in the interstitium as well as within the lumens of distal tubules (fig. 53). Charcot used the term "uric acid infarcts" to describe

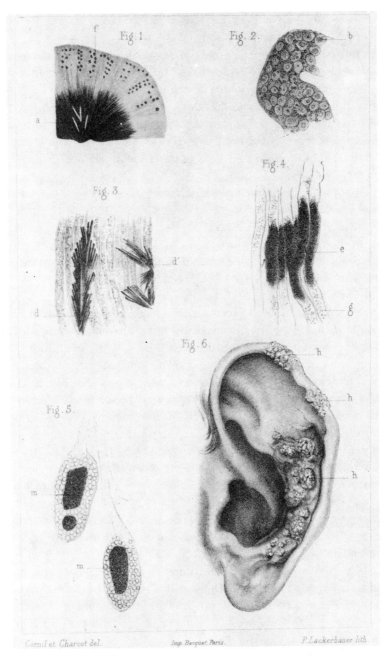

53. *Jean-Martin Charcot in 1864 was the first to illustrate histologic detail of the gouty kidney. Figure 1 shows medullary streaks of uric acid while figure 4 shows their origin in the lumens of distal tubules. Charcot termed the cortical microtophi (black dots in fig. 1) "uric acid infarcts" (127).*

the microtophi, emphasizing their similarity to vascular obstructions but obscuring their pathogenesis.

By the end of the nineteenth century, the distinguishing features of gouty nephropathy were remembered by few. Nevertheless, in 1883, J. Milner Fothergill, who counted among his credits an honorary medical degree from the Rush Medical School and an associate fellowship of the College of Physicians in Philadelphia, wrote of proteinuria, "It is not the common associate of gout nor is it usually found with the gouty kidney" (268, p. 26). In America the views of this London physician were honored less than was he.

In 1950, John Talbott included renal failure or calculi as two of the four major clinical criteria for the diagnosis of gout (727). Although nonspecific interstitial nephritis was recognized as the typical renal lesion of gout in the nineteenth century (533, 767), some modern investigators seem to have convinced themselves that unique glomerular and tubular lesions are present (312, 824).

Current classifications of renal disease in gout usually list three mechanisms of organ damage: 1) renal calculus, 2) acute intratubular crystal deposition, and 3) gouty nephropathy (80). The first two conditions are commonly encountered in uric acid excess with or without gout. These forms of renal disease appear to be independent of direct lead nephrotoxicity.

The term "gouty nephropathy" had been used to designate a variety of renal diseases some of which are probably unrelated to gout. Proteinuric renal disease (glomerulonephritis) has frequently been confused with gouty nephropathy (73, 95, 100, 155, 260, 329, 342, 496, 522, 531, 584, 674). It seems likely that one reason for the confusion of primary glomerular disease with gout nephropathy has been the ease with which proteinuria is detected in the clinical laboratory. But urinary protein excretion increases as renal failure progresses, regardless of the underlying cause (47). Once the end stage of renal disease is reached, valid etiologic differentiation is often impossible (100, 428, 496, 674).

Innumerable mechanisms for the production of interstitial nephritis in gout have been hypothesized. The idea that renal damage is induced by uric acid remains convincing to many students of this subject (272, 688), but whether the deposits are a consequence of interstitial nephritis or its cause is unsettled (80, 413).

While crystal deposition undoubtedly contributes to renal failure, there is no evidence that such deposits are the sole or major cause of interstitial nephritis when no crystals are present. Nor is it clear how focal deposits induce interstitial disease throughout the kidney. There is, moreover, reason to suspect that urate deposition in the interstitial space may be a secondary phenomenon comparable to urate deposition in other connective tissues throughout the body (42, 413).

Recently an experimental model of gouty nephropathy has been developed in rats which supports the view that extreme hyperuricemia per se is sometimes responsible for interstitial nephritis (73, 424). Rats fed the uricase inhibitor oxonic acid are unable to break down uric acid which then accumulates in their blood. Renal failure characterized by intraluminal crystal deposition rapidly ensues. If the rats survive for up to a year, interstitial nephritis develops. But despite the similarity of the intratubular crystal deposition to classic descriptions of the gouty kidney, this model of uric acid nephropathy is more akin to acute intraluminal obstruction than to chronic interstitial nephritis of long-standing gout (699). Intratubular crystal deposition in rats occurs at a far lower serum uric acid level than in man and the vascular changes found in gouty kidneys are conspicuously absent (424). Very similar lesions have been produced in animals by intravenous infusions of lithium urate (207, 208). However, there has been a tendency to assume that interstitial nephritis consequent to acute intraluminal crystal deposition is identical to that occurring in the absence of observable crystal deposits. This assumption makes it difficult, if not unnecessary, to identify other mechanisms of production of interstitial nephritis in gout.

Recurring reports of uric acid deposits in kidneys of patients who had no history of gout have brought the significance of intrarenal crystal deposits into question (15, 100, 117, 204, 391, 575, 635, 763). Uric acid deposition appears to be a late event in chronic renal failure unrelated to gout; microtophi have been found in kidneys of patients with lead nephropathy who never had acute articular disease (391). As usual, the frequency of such findings depends on the investigator's eagerness to make the observation (234). The contention that renal microtophi are specific for gout (692, 695, 728, 796) would appear to be untenable. Although hyperuricemia is universal in renal failure, gout is distinctly unusual in uremic patients (551). Histologically, it is obvious that the interstitial pathology is not limited to areas of the kidney in which crystals are present. If the deposits are secondary, local, and benign, the question arises as to whether urate deposition should be considered at all a cause of widespread interstitial nephritis.

In birds, nitrogenous waste products are normally excreted as uric acid. This is analagous to the excretion of urea in mammalian urine. Despite the relatively huge amount of uric acid which is excreted by the avian kidney, urate-induced renal disease is rare. In birds, then, hyperuricemia does not appear to be nephrotoxic. In certain avian strains, however, massive deposition of urate is sometimes found throughout the body—a syndrome reminiscent of "irregular gout" and not inappropriately called "visceral gout" (686). Although there is no joint involvement in these birds, the kidneys are severely damaged. In view of the ability of birds to excrete relatively enormous quantities of uric acid without difficulty, the appearance of urate nephropathy in birds is regarded as the result of, rather than the cause of, renal disease. The renal disease reduces urate excretion and leads to widespread uratic precipitates in the viscera including the kidney.

The current trend to avoid treating asymptomatic hyperuricemia in patients with renal failure attests to a growing conviction that modest elevations of serum uric acid are not damaging to the kidneys (234, 255, 630). The antihyperuricemic agent, allopurinol, has been shown to have little or no beneficial effect on the gouty kidney (85, 94, 237, 305, 458, 559, 638, 656, 787). Nevertheless, the question of when to use allopurinol in asymptomatic patients remains a subject of controversy (707, 811).

In the absence of intra- or extrarenal obstruction or urate deposits in the kidney, the pathogenesis of the interstitial nephritis of gout is particularly puzzling. In 1864, Danjoy first suggested that this renal disease might in fact sometimes be due to lead, an idea that won few adherents (178). Yet the first published illustration of the histopathology of the gouty kidney (fig. 54), was strikingly similar to the renal histology of saturnine gout seen by Lancereaux (fig. 55), to the lead nephropathy seen by Oliver (fig. 46), and to that seen in contemporary renal biopsies (fig. 56). Lancereaux's illustration was from the kidney of a ship painter who suffered colic, palsy, and gout during life and died of interstitial nephritis (438).

The gouty kidney was also widely recognized in England after Garrod's observations (512), but the fact that lead by itself could induce renal disease was less generally appreciated (453). Commenting on Garrod's lead workers with gout, Basham wrote in 1870 (45): "Can we, then, regard lead as exercising any specific effect on the kidneys? I think not, except so far as susceptibility to gout does so. In every case of albuminous urine occurring in painters that I have seen there has been evidence of gouty attacks" (p. 28). The view thus evolved that gout increased susceptibility to lead nephropathy rather than the reverse (653).

Although lead became accepted as a cause of both gout and kidney dis-

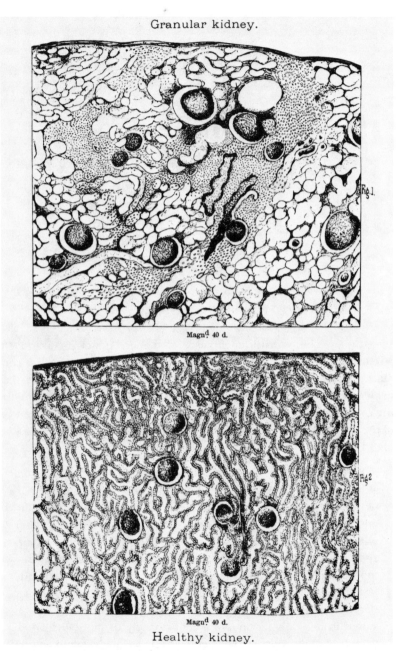

Granular kidney.

Magn^d 40 d.

Magn^d 40 d.

Healthy kidney.

54. *This illustration of interstitial nephritis in gout by Dickinson in 1881 (190) shows neither crystals nor inflammatory cell infiltrates (above). Compare to normal renal histology (below).*

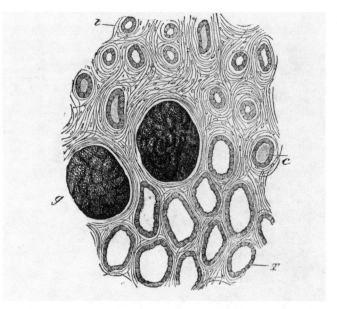

55. *Interstitial nephritis in saturnine kidney illustrated by Lancereaux in 1872 (438).*

ease, the possibility that it might also cause gouty kidney received little attention. In 1868, William Dickinson drew this not unreasonable conclusion (189). In contrast to glomerulonephritis, Dickinson noted that urine was usually free of albumin, and that polyuria was more common at the onset than oliguria. Of forty-five patients with granular degeneration of the kidney, Dickinson found that ten had past evidence of lead poisoning (190).

From these particulars it is not too much to assert that of painters at least one half eventually die of granular degeneration of the kidneys; while as compared to other external circumstances the influence of lead is a more fertile source of this disease than any other with which we are acquainted. . . . The gout affection of the joints and granular degeneration are associated as springing from a common cause. If the morbid tendency affect the joints we have the ordinary symptoms of gout; if the kidney, the characteristic granular degeneration. It appears that where the gouty condition has resulted from alcoholic liquors it tends chiefly to the joints; when from lead to the kidneys. The rich man enjoys long life with gout in his extremities, the artisan perishes before his limbs are touched, from change of the same nature in the kidney (p. 110).

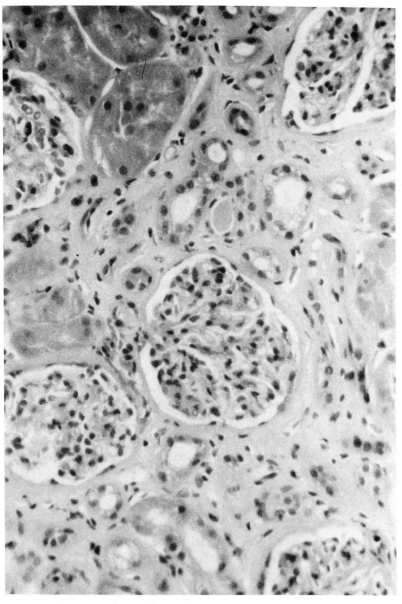

56. Lead nephropathy in an asymptomatic lead worker, 1975.

Lancereaux concurred in this explanation. "The nephritis and arthritis of saturnism," he affirmed in 1881, "are precisely the identical lesions of the nephritis and arthritis of gout" (439, p. 652).

The increased frequency of renal disease in saturnine gout as opposed to nonlead gout was impressive. In 1875, Lecorché noted (449), "Saturnine gout is distinguished from ordinary gout in that the urate deposits, instead of occurring around the joints, occur in the kidneys" (p. 368).

In 1886, Lorimer could find few distinctions between lead and nonlead gout, but concluded, "Gout associated with lead impregnation, however, seems to attack the kidneys" (476, p. 163). Duckworth reported that 18 percent of his patients with gout "presented signs of lead impregnation, and followed the occupation of painters, plumbers, compositors or workers in lead mills" (204, p. 152). He uniformly found interstitial nephritis in these patients.

It is curious that such keen observers as Garrod and Charcot, both intimately involved in the initial descriptions of saturnine gout, overlooked the possible common etiology. In retrospect a number of circumstances may have obscured the relationship. First, renal disease was detected primarily by proteinuria. Consequently, only advanced interstitial nephritis was discovered. Second, pathologic examinations were restricted to postmortem specimens. The gouty kidney was seen histologically only at the end point of the disease. Third, lead intoxication was diagnosed by overt symptomatology; chronic low-level absorption or exposure in the remote past did not present the hallmarks of acute lead intoxication. Finally, the effects of uric acid and lead on the kidney were clouded by the frequent coexistence of hypertension and urinary tract infection. Both Garrod and Charcot shared the contemporary view that gout was a systemic disease. Charcot taught that gout of the stomach was often fatal. Like Garrod, he remained uncertain about the role of lead. "It now remains to determine the cause of this singular coincidence," he mused in 1881 (130, p. 90). Uncertainty in the minds of these influential physicians overshadowed the interpretations of less renowned observers.

German physicians remained aloof to the controversies surrounding gout generated in England and France until the end of the nineteenth century. The first German review of the subject appeared in 1896 by H. Luthje (480). After chastising his compatriots for neglecting the subject, Luthje documented the case for saturnine gout. "It is the renal atrophy," he concluded, "which makes saturnine gout lethal" (p. 306). Explaining why epidemiologic surveys failed to identify the syndrome, Luthje stated, "The victim of lead poisoning gives up his occupation at an early age due to the various maladies from which he suffers—or he may die of one of the lead conditions (possibly nephritis) before the gout has an opportunity to develop" (p. 295). The vagaries of epidemiologic studies were not unique to Luthje's time or place.

Confusion about the role of lead was further promoted by the conviction that alcohol itself caused kidney damage. Alcohol was considered the cause of kidney disease as well as of colic, gout, and encephalopathy. In 1836 Richard Bright expressed the view that, next to scarlatina, drunkenness was the most common cause of chronic renal disease. He did not suspect that lead rather than alcohol might be responsible for this association. "A more impressive warning against the intemperate use of ardent spirits," he wrote, "cannot be derived from any other form of disease with which we are acquainted" (93, p. 339). Echoing the precepts espoused by Bright, Basham went further. "Intemperance brings more victims to chronic renal disease," this early nephrologist asserted, "than all the other causes put together" (45, p. 157).

In the moral climate of the growing temperance movement, blaming drunkenness was comfortable (54, 143, 314). The idea that immorality contributed to the demise of the gouty was consistent with theological teaching and popular gossip. The traditional view gained credibility from scientific observation. Physicians had, once again, found exactly what they were seeking; intemperance met its just reward and the convictions of the pious were vindicated.

The allegory of gout was depicted in the title page of a 1623 tract on podagra (fig. 57). Scenes at the top and along the sides illustrate the luxurious existence—the pleasures of the hunt enlivened with wine, women, and song. The consequences of licentious living are depicted in the lower panels; a gouty old man hobbles on crutches, surrounded by Venus and Bacchus. In the final panel, our debauchee is bedridden, a terminal case. The wages of sin is death. On his deathbed the invalid is accompanied only by a uroscopist, attempting to forecast his sad fate from the urine (788). Gout was the occupational disease of the libertine, and death from renal failure the sure reward.

Alcohol was believed to cause the shrunken granular kidneys found at postmortem examination. Edema and proteinuria, if they occurred at all, were late or terminal manifestations of the renal disease of intemperance. In contrast, scarlatina was associated with large white kidneys following rapidly fatal acute glomerulonephritis. These patients did not survive long enough to develop contracted kidneys. In a later epoch, physicians learned to prevent death from infection and fluid retention in the acute

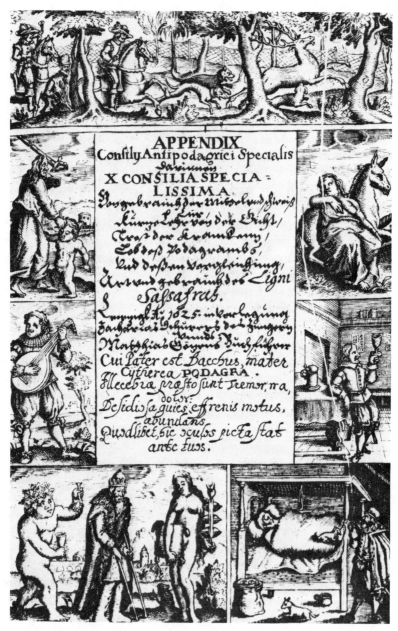

57. On his death-bed, in this 1623 illustration, the gouty debauchee finds that
Bacchus and Venus have been replaced by a dog and uroscopist (582).

phase of poststreptococcal glomerulonephritis. The large white kidney, also called lardaceous or waxy, is now rarely encountered at postmortem.

The English did not share Ollivier's suspicion that renal disease in alcoholics was perhaps due to lead exposure (568). And so for some physicians, at least, lead nephropathy was due to gout or alcohol (54, 453) and interstitial nephritis was defined by albuminuria or stones. The interaction of multiple causes of renal disease served to obscure the separate characteristics of each. To dissect the role of lead in gout and gouty nephropathy seemed hopeless (247), possibly because of the absence of a method for assessing body lead stores.

The Contemporary View

Given the uncertainty of the masters of pathologic anatomy, it is perhaps no wonder that their successors became increasingly unsure about the role of lead in kidney disease. The important distinction between proteinuric and nonproteinuric renal disease was often missed. It is almost impossible to determine from published descriptions whether the renal disease described was due to nonspecific end-stage kidneys, incidental glomerular disease, or interstitial nephritis.

Confusion concerning the specific causes of renal disease was compounded in 1939 by Weiss and Parker's description of bacterial invasion of the kidneys, healed "pyelonephritis" (42, 100, 312, 461, 728, 778, 797). Weiss and Parker recognized that etiology could not be determined by histology alone, but should be based on clinical evidence of renal infection (797). However, they never specified the critical clinical diagnostic criteria. They accepted nephrosclerosis and hypertension as a consequence of "pyelonephritis" but failed to resolve the question of other possible causes of similar histopathology. "In connection with this group of chronic pyelonephritis," these experts contended, "cases of so called interstitial nephritis must be mentioned. . . . this type of lesion represents chronic or healed pyelonephritis" (p. 238).

A variety of indirect bits of evidence were developed to support the hypothesis that "interstitial nephritis" was due to bacterial invasion of the kidney; X-ray findings, immunohistology, circulating antibodies, and bacterial coating by antibodies were cited in support of the Weiss and Parker concept. According to this view, renal parenchymal infection could be identified in the absence of viable bacteria in the tissue.

While bacterial invasion of the kidney is common in the presence of ureteral obstruction, acceptance of the diagnosis of infection without bacteriologic proof obscured other causes of interstitial nephritis for decades. When the frequency of pyelonephritis was reviewed in university hospitals in the United States, the incidence determined from postmortem examinations varied a thousandfold—from 0.2 to 20 percent (370). This enormous variability could best be explained by divergent diagnostic criteria. Pathologists who accepted the Weiss and Parker thesis frequently diagnosed chronic pyelonephritis, while more critical authors rarely accepted that diagnosis. The assumption that infected urine indicated progressive renal parenchymal disease was severely weakened by subsequent studies of urinary tract infection without obstruction (274). The idea that urinary tract infection caused renal disease in the absence of anatomical abnormalities of the urinary tract could not be substantiated (273).

"Healed pyelonephritis" failed to withstand close scrutiny (17). As in centuries past, modern physicians, under enormous pressure to find surcease for human suffering, are tempted to accept hypothesis as fact. Physicians find it difficult to acknowledge their ignorance. Despite impressive evidence for the existence of lead nephropathy, this diagnosis was rejected in favor of "pyelonephritis."

The semantic confusion surrounding "pyelonephritis" was doubly troublesome in gout. Ancient writers had referred to acute ureteral obstruction and the attendant renal symptoms as "nephritis." It is just this type of obstruction with infection which is still considered bona fide pyelonephritis (bacterial invasion of the renal parenchyma). By terming both nonbacterial interstitial nephritis and bacterial invasion "pyelonephritis," separation of these entities became impossible.

Hypertension and gout, long associated with lead poisoning, have further confounded recognition of lead nephropathy (42, 52, 53, 64, 89, 334, 340, 352, 427, 443, 501, 502, 526, 527, 534–40, 562, 578, 579, 584, 636, 673, 766). Some observers have not found gout (37, 468, 632, 728, 729, 761) or hypertension (57, 91, 164, 269, 508, 520, 622) in association with lead poisoning while others have noted a consistent association (29, 191, 227–38, 286, 368, 398, 453, 476, 534–40, 564, 594, 636, 766).

The connection of hypertension with both gout and lead poisoning was described even before a clinically practical method for measuring blood pressure was available. Richard Bright had noted that the heart was usually enlarged in patients who died of kidney disease. It was assumed that cardiac enlargement was a consequence of the metabolic abnormalities of uremia until Gull and Sutton observed that death from chronic renal failure could occur with a normal size heart (340, 341). The mechanism whereby the kidney affected the heart was unclear until F. A. Mahomed, successor to Richard Bright at Guy's Hospital, found that a "long and hard" pulse was the most frequent sign of renal disease. Using a sphygmograph devised by Burdon-Sanderson in 1867 to record arterial pulse tracings, he noted that hypertension often preceded clinical manifestations of both kidney and heart failure (501, 502). Mahomed concluded that hypertension was the major cause of the granular kidney.

Mahomed recognized the perennial dilemma of determining whether hypertension causes the renal disease or renal disease causes the hypertension. Vascular changes indicative of hypertension are typically found in nonhypertensive gouty kidneys just as they are in lead nephropathy (80, 100, 391, 584, 793). Moreover, the kidney in hypertension shows anatomic changes indistinguishable from interstitial nephritis (391). Eventually, Mahomed came to believe that vascular disease was primary and that the term "arteriocapillary fibrosis," proposed by Gull and Sutton, should replace the term "interstitial nephritis" (503). He included the gouty kidney in this designation, but believed plumbism was more often the result of the treatment of renal disease than its cause.

The primacy of vascular abnormalities as the cause of kidney disease gained many adherents (177, 405, 406, 452). In the Harvey Lectures of 1912, Theodore Janeway expressed the view that hypertensive vascular disease of the kidney is a consequence of exogenous toxins. "One poison," he asserted, "which in rare cases produces acute gout, is the single cause of cardiovascular disease upon which we can definitely put our fingers. That poison is lead" (398, p. 236). To complicate the matter further, the transient vascular spasm associated with acute lead colic (38, 562, 617, 761, 769) was sometimes confused with the persistent structural renal vascular damage noted in chronic lead exposure. The similarity of the histologic features of hypertensive kidney to that of interstitial nephritis was so strong that it was suggested that the term "nephrosclerosis" or "arteriosclerotic hypertensive kidney" replace "interstitial nephritis" (717). Association confounded causation and semantics compounded the problem.

The pathogenesis of vascular alterations in lead nephropathy is as obscure as in essential hypertension. It is uncertain which comes first, tubular damage, nephrosclerosis, or interstitial disease (410, 595). As noted by Nye, "It is almost a matter of coincidence whether the syndrome is called arteriosclerosis, hypertension, etc., or chronic nephritis" (557).

Hypertension is one of the concomitants of plumbism that has withstood reassessment in the twentieth century (47, 89, 118, 256, 403, 789, 790). Evidence that high blood pressure is a consequence of plumbism naturally raised the question whether hypertension in gout patients might have the same origin. Rapado recently investigated the possibility that the hypertension associated with gout is a consequence of insidious lead absorption. He found that a history of lead exposure was five times more common among gout patients with hypertension than in those with normal blood pressures (623). In the hypertensive, uric acid excretion was lower and renal disease more common; but the causal relationships, based solely on the patient's recall of past exposure, remained uncertain. Had the EDTA test been used in evaluating these 750 gout patients, far more convincing separation of lead and nonlead groups might have been achieved.

In a recent survey of subjects exposed to lead in drinking water, elevated blood lead concentrations were found along with increased serum uric acid and urea nitrogen concentrations. Elevated blood lead values predicted the presence of hypertension, gout, and early renal failure (52, 53, 114) despite the absence of the classical symptoms of lead poisoning.

Intensive investigation of the metabolic and hormonal changes associated with high blood pressure have provided little compelling information concerning the etiology of essential hypertension. Contemporary studies, molded by available technology and the demand for therapy, may be focused on the secondary and tertiary consequences of high blood pressure, while more mundane pathogenic mechanisms are all but ignored. The possibility exists, for example, that alterations in plasma renin and aldosterone levels found in some hypertensive patients might be mediated by lead. There is evidence that lead induces hyporeninemic hypoaldosteronism in association with hypertension in both man and experimental animals (313, 483, 537, 667). But contradictory reports have also been filed (113). Unexpected elevations of the serum potassium concentration in gout patients might similarly be related to an underlying and unsuspected lead etiology (259). Direct effects on sodium-potassium ATPase (239, 412) and on kallikrein production by the kidney (142) are also being explored to explain the hypertension of chronic plumbism, but have not yet found general acceptance.

In order to determine if unrecognized excessive lead absorption might account for the renal disease in some hypertensives, we recently examined patients at the Veterans Administration Medical Center in East Orange, New Jersey. The results suggested that lead was responsible for renal impairment in many (46). Lead excretion during the three-day EDTA lead-mobilization test was significantly greater in hypertensives with renal failure than in hypertensives with normal renal function. The hypertensives also excreted more lead than patients with comparable renal failure of other known etiologies. Since these men had never had symptoms of lead intoxication, the lead mobilization test would not normally have been performed and their hypertension would have been deemed "essential." The hypertensives with renal disease also differed from those without renal failure in that the duration of their high blood pressure averaged only seven years compared to fourteen years in those with preserved renal function. This finding contradicts the hypothesis that the renal failure was a consequence of prolonged hypertension. Our finding of excessive lead in hypertensive men with renal disease suggests that lead may sometimes be the cause of renal failure in "essential" hypertension. The findings also raise the possibility that unrecognized lead absorption may contribute to the high frequency of hypertension progressing to end-stage renal disease in blacks as compared to whites.

One conceivable mechanism that could relate high blood pressure and insidious lead poisoning is immunologic. Lead has been shown to modify the immune response in mice (429, 430). The possibility that immune processes may sometimes be responsible for hypertensive vascular disease has been raised in a number of recent studies (216, 339, 548, 569). In patients with occupational lead nephropathy, renal biopsy specimens showed a surprising degree of antibody deposition (794). Perhaps immune mechanisms are the common ground upon which the renal disease of both hypertension and lead nephropathy progress. The identification of immunoglobulins in the kidneys, however, by no means proves the pathogenic mechanism. In conjunction with the observation that nephrosclerosis is often seen in lead nephropathy patients in the *absence* of hypertension, the hypothesis that both hypertension and interstitial nephritis are mediated by immunologic mechanisms, nevertheless, seems tenable. Immunologic abnormalities triggered by lead could account for the presence of hypertension and interstitial nephritis in both gout and lead nephropathy (789, 790).

A more direct nephrotoxic effect has been observed in those rare circumstances in which lead has been administered intravenously. In marked contrast to the nephropathy induced by chronic low-dose lead absorption, this form of lead nephropathy is characterized by acute tubular necrosis and the rapid development of uremia. Death occurs within days or weeks unless dialytic substitutes for kidney function are pro-

212 · Poison in the Pot

vided. If the acute renal failure is survived, the kidneys often spontaneously recover as in other forms of acute tubular necrosis.

It is now widely recognized that urate deposition in kidneys may be only a late manifestation of gouty nephropathy (424). Talbott has observed that "since only a small percentage of kidneys in gouty patients have urate deposits the term gouty kidney should not depend on the finding of urate crystals in the kidney" (728, p. 409). Although he noted the similarity between the renal histology of gout and lead poisoning, Talbott reported that only 4 of 279 gouty patients with postmortem kidney examinations were known to have worked with lead. In describing the hematologic causes of gout, Talbott accepted lead workers as having saturnine gout only if they had anemia, colic, constipation, and wrist drop. In men with less flagrant symptomatology, he was uncertain of the role of lead in eliciting gout, despite the presence of anemia and stippled red cells. Talbott did not consider lead an important cause of gout because of the absence of acute lead poisoning. In 1957 he wrote, "The widespread use of this heavy metal and the low incidence of gout among exposed workers suggest no causal relationship" (725, p. 116).

Talbott failed to distinguish between the various causes of renal disease (727). Pooling a spectrum of renal diseases he reported that "albuminuria, the presence of white or red blood cells and casts in the urinary sediment, impaired concentrating ability, mild nitrogen retention, even abnormal pyelography have been observed singly or together in approximately 50% of our series" (728, p. 454). These manifold problems he attributed to gout.

The American view of nephropathy in gout was summarized by Wyngaarden and Kelly in 1976 (822).

> Chronic renal disease is the second most common manifestation of gout. Progressive renal failure currently accounts for 17 to 25 percent of the deaths in the gouty population. . . .
>
> A common manifestation of urate nephropathy is albuminuria which occurs in 20 to 40 percent of patients with gout. A history of gouty arthritis suggests that urate nephropathy may be the underlying disease, since gout is rare in chronic renal failure of other etiologies and the extent of urate nephropathy is usually correlated with the severity of gouty arthritis (p. 242).

In an earlier publication citing the same incidence of proteinuria, Wyngaarden pointed out that the incidence of hypertension was also 20 to 40 percent in patients with gout. Among their many other distinctions, John H. Talbott is a former editor of *The Journal of the American Medical Association* and present editor of *Seminars in Arthritis and Rheumatism* and James B. Wyngaarden is currently director of the National Institutes of Health. Their immense influence on medical thinking is not easily controverted.

Conventional concepts of gouty nephropathy (80, 822, 824) do not require recognition of a subclass of interstitial nephritis in gout which is slowly progressive, nonglomerular, and independent of urate deposition. In the United States over the last fifty years, descriptions of gouty nephropathy have usually omitted reference to the role of lead (39, 48, 80, 155, 312, 329). In the absence of microtophi, the interstitial nephritis has either been ignored or attributed to "a reaction of the kidney to an increased filtered load of urate or some, as yet unidentified precursor, analagous to what is seen in hypercalcemic nephropathy" (312, p. 672). Even when lead has been considered a possible cause of gout, it has not been suspected as a possible cause of gouty nephropathy (478, 576, 674, 822). Nevertheless, lead exposure continues to be associated with hyperuricemia, hypertension, and renal failure (53, 114, 116).

In 1975, Berger and Yü challenged the basic tenets of gouty nephropathy. They reported that hyperuricemia and gout do not result in renal disease even after many years (62). Meticulous renal function studies in 624 gout patients followed by Yü and Berger for over two decades at the Mt. Sinai Hospital in New York led these workers to conclude that renal failure in gout is due to hypertension, vascular disease, or unrelated renal disease rather than to hyperuricemia (823–25).

There is no reason to believe that the Mt. Sinai gout patients without hypertension or renal failure, if properly tested, would show excessive lead absorption. EDTA testing, of those *with* renal failure might provide very different results, however. It would not be surprising if the renal failure group showed excessive mobilizable lead consistent with saturnine gout, but the incidence of gout among patients at Mt. Sinai Hospital would be expected to be lower than at a Veterans Administration Hospital. The middle-class patients seen at Mt. Sinai Hospital with uncomplicated gout may have far less exposure to lead than Englishmen of a former era or modern armed services veterans. Life-style could then be considered the critical determinant of the gouty kidney. The Mt. Sinai findings are supported by observations made in San Francisco, London, and Glasgow which show that chronic renal disease does not develop in hyperuricemic patients even after many years (255–57, 304, 622). The absence of gouty nephropathy in these very large series of patients followed for decades contradicts the medical dictum that gout ends in renal failure.

The rarity of lead poisoning among certain groups in the United States may account for the gradual disappearance of renal disease in gout. The socioeconomic base of saturnine gout has been emphasized by Gene Ball (40). "How common is saturnine gout?" he asked rhetorically. "In my private practice I have never seen a case; in the VA Hospital [in Birmingham, Alabama] gout is almost always saturnine" (p. 283). This anecdotal experience has recently gained scientific support from a national survey of blood leads among ten thousand citizens (500). Lower socioeconomic groups consistently show high blood levels, the highest being found in poor, black, male children. This early exposure to lead may contribute to the excessive incidence of hypertension with severe renal failure found later in life in black men (479).

The hypothesis that some patients with renal disease and gout have unrecognized lead nephropathy resolves a number of the most tenacious controversies in medicine. Lead could account for the ancient association of gout with colic, palsy, and cerebral disease ("irregular gout"). It may also explain the long and controversial association with wine and the variable incidence of gout. Most important, lead can account for progressive interstitial nephritis in certain gout populations.

To test this hypothesis, we examined forty-four veterans with gout in East Orange, New Jersey, for possible excessive body lead stores using the EDTA lead-mobilization test. Excessive chelatable lead was found in thirteen of twenty-two with renal failure but in only four of twenty-two gout patients with normal renal function. None of the veterans had ever experienced symptoms of lead poisoning. The severity of renal disease varied directly with the mobilizable lead (47, 739), a finding which has also been observed in occupational lead nephropathy (790). These results suggest that lead may, indeed, explain the conflicting experiences with gouty nephropathy over the last century.

The source of the excessive stores of lead in the New Jersey veterans is far from clear, although a history of moonshine consumption was common whether or not the gout was associated with renal failure. But these men also had frequent exposure to lead in transient work situations. The contribution of lead in the environment is also problematic. Both gasoline residues and lead contamination of food are ubiquitous in modern urban life. A recent assessment of lead in canned food demonstrated a forty thousandfold increase in the lead in tuna fish from prehistoric to modern times (681). The only conclusion that can reasonably be drawn from our data with respect to the source of exposure is that patients do not know when or where they absorb lead. Patients' recollections do not jibe with the objective evidence of the EDTA lead-mobilization test. Our findings seem to support Charcot's statement of 1878 (128): "The gout of saturnine subjects, from what I have seen, appears to differ from ordinary gout only in the greater rapidity of its evolution, the abundance of to-phaceous deposits, and the necessary existence, so to term it, of renal lesions" (p. 65).

The excessive lead in our patients with gout or hypertension and renal failure provides evidence of the role of lead in these nephropathies. Lead seems to be responsible for the renal disease in these patients because control patients with comparable renal failure did not have excess mobilizable lead. The conclusion is based on the assumption that renal dysfunction in the control patients was comparable with respect to lead metabolism to that in the hypertensive and gout patients. Since the mean serum creatinines were not significantly different, the assumption seems valid. On the other hand, the control patients had either glomerular or systemic disease—conditions necessary to assure an accurate diagnosis of renal disease *not* due to lead or gout. Tubular function or bone metabolism could, however, conceivably by systematically different in the control group. Measurements of bone lead in uremic and dialysis patients have not shown any increase in lead stores (44, 235, 369, 391, 675, 790), nor does renal failure by itself reduce urinary lead excretion (115). While there is, therefore, at present no reason to believe that differences in lead metabolism exist between groups of renal failure patients, this possibility will be difficult to exclude completely until more is known about the cause and course of chronic renal failure. It should be noted that even if such unlikely disparities existed, they would have no bearing on occupational lead nephropathy.

Despite the support of history, histology, and therapeutic response, the possibility of ubiquitous lead nephropathy seems incredible to many (824). The idea that "normal" blood levels may be dangerous is contrary to their experience. To support the preconception that no such danger exists, scientists attack the selection of controls and hypothesize that renal failure causes excessive mobilizable lead rather than the reverse. Experts are reluctant to believe that they have overlooked something fundamental in their area of expertise. In a recent study from the moonshine belt, the authors resorted to statistical gyrations in order to obscure the fact that the EDTA lead-mobilization test had identified lead as the unrecognized cause of renal dysfunction in their gout patients (633). In another report showing two elevated EDTA tests among nine gout patients with renal failure, it was concluded that lead is unimportant in the production of renal disease in gout (670).

The suspicion that lead causes more renal disease than has previously been recognized seems conservative, however, compared to the views of Clair Patterson. Pattersons's studies of human lead production and its geophysical dispersion have led him to conclude that enough information is already at hand to warrant bringing to a "halt the mining and smelting of lead and the manufacturing of leaded products within the shortest possible time" (546, p. 272). In Patterson's view, everyone suffers the ill effects of lead, not just a few subpopulations who are clinically defined. Having reduced the accepted "normal" value for lead in preindustrial man a thousandfold using exquisitely sensitive, ultraclean, isotope dilution mass spectroscopy, Patterson finds the complacency of responsible officialdom incredible. Bone lead concentrations are twenty to one hundred times greater in modern than in prehistoric man (202, 322, 323). The importance of this fact is consigned to a minority opinion, written by Patterson, and attached to the report on *Lead in the Human Environment* prepared by the National Academy of Sciences in 1980 (546). It should be noted that Patterson is concerned with the lowest level of detectable lead—a million times less than is found in the urine during EDTA testing of lead nephropathy patients.

Lead nephrotoxicity represents a relatively high level of asymptomatic absorption in man rather than the lowest. The renal findings warrant only one conclusion in common with Patterson's; as long as inadequate techniques are employed to investigate the toxicologic impact of lead, committee decisions will be equivocal and demands for vaguely conceived reinvestigations numerous. Controversy will not be resolved by even a geometric increase in the already astronomical literature on lead without considerably more attention being paid to methodologic detail.

The history of lead and the kidney suggests that lead nephropathy in its several manifestations was obscured for a century because the right questions were not raised. This jigsaw puzzle, largely pieced together by 1870, was disassembled over the next few decades. The keys to the dissolution were to be found in the past. George Baker and Tanquerel des Planches had failed to recognize saturnine gout, nephropathy, or hypertension. Bright's disease, of fundamental importance to the development of scientific medicine in the nineteenth century, was operationally defined by the presence of proteinuria. Lacking proteinuria in its early phases, interstitial nephritis received little attention, and was further confounded by misleading language. As long as lead poisoning was defined by the classical acute symptoms of colic followed by the palsy, even the addition of hematologic abnormalities to the diagnostic criteria did not permit detection of chronic low dose lead exposure.

If the analysis of history and clinical data presented in this book is correct, perhaps we can look forward to a renewed interest in the biologic consequences of lead. A new formulation of questions will surely elicit compelling answers for the future. The outlook then, is that of the College of Physicians of London when George Baker published his observations on the Devonshire colic in the first volume of the *Medical Transactions* in 1768. The new journal began with some sanguine reflections, echoing Sir Francis Bacon, which are valid for all such beginnings (213).

The experience of many ages hath more than sufficiently shewn, that mere abstract reasonings have tended very little to the promoting of natural knowledge. By laying these aside, and attending carefully to what nature hath either by chance or upon experiment offered to our observation, a greater progress hath been made in this part of philosophy, since the beginning of the last century, than had been till that time from the days of Aristotle.

Epilogue

The legacy of lead consists of overt and insidious poisoning for mankind from prehistoric times to the present. The historical trail is strewn with frustrated attempts to control and prevent this disease, which follows in the tracks of human ingenuity. Warnings, supported by hard scientific evidence, have fostered irregular progress over the millennia. The redundancy of the alarms has, perhaps, inured the public to the dangers lurking downwind of smelters and in epicurean repasts. Physicians have undermined their own authority by complacency, if not arrogance, while merchants and manufacturers have shown a careless greed throughout the conflict. When the issue has been joined, economic and health interests have clashed. "Cost-benefit" has been the battlefield, but whose "cost," and whose "benefit," never clearly stated. The combat has been fought with words obscured by ambiguity and conflicting goals. The choice between work and health presents a perpetual dilemma (549).

Following publication of his *Treatise on Adulterations of Food, and Culinary Poisons* in 1820, Fredrick Accum was stunned by the anger his revelations incurred. In the preface to his second edition, he met the threats of anonymous critics with defiance. Of those who would suppress his work, Accum wrote, "Their menaces will in no way prevent me from endeavoring to put the unwary on their guard against the frauds of dishonest men, wherever they may originate; and those assailants in ambush are hereby informed, that, in every succeeding edition of the work, I shall continue to hand down to posterity the infamy which justly attaches to the knaves and dishonest dealers, who have been convicted at the bar of Public Justice for rendering human food deleterious to health" (1, pp. x–xi). Accum was careful to mention by name only those manufacturers whose misdeeds were already cited in the public record. With the establishment of the Food and Drug Administration in the United States, this adversary stance has shifted to the arena of industrial and environmental health.

In modern times, plebeian workmen have replaced the Roman aristocracy as the major victims of unrecognized plumbism. The fruit of man's labor has displaced the fruit of the vine as the focus of concern. Physicians remain key combatants on both sides of the fray, but their attention has shifted from colic, palsy, and the gout to the delayed effects on brain and kidney. It is these organs which appear to be the critical targets of chronic low-level lead absorption.

Despite its lack of romance, the kidney may prove of fundamental importance in assessing the hazards of lead. The ability to measure renal function with precision provides solid evidence, in contrast to the relatively soft data from behavioral studies. End-stage renal disease programs throughout the world have brought kidney disease into sharp focus. The cost of dialysis and transplantation attracts more attention than pathophysiologic constructions. The threads of past knowledge are now being picked up, and earlier concepts of renal disease are being reexamined. Pressure for diagnostic precision is generated by the need for prevention (791).

Environmental lead contamination is not likely to be eliminated until there is much broader comprehension of its consequences. Federal regulators are in a position to increase public awareness, but it is difficult for politically sensitive institutions to assign blame or initiate reform. The Environmental Protection Agency has codified the evidence incriminating lead in the production of renal disease (239). Lead seems to be accountable where gout or hypertension were previously blamed. When the victims realize that liability for their plight can be established, the civil courts will hear their complaints and juries will respond sympathetically. Monetary awards against the manufacturers will assure corrective action as no plodding bureaucracy can. The insurance companies will see to it that the workplace is made safe.

The successful law suit by asbestos workers against the Manville Corporation established a precedent. It remains only for creative lawyers to process the liability claims of victims of lead nephropathy now languishing among the ever growing population of renal dialysis patients. In the past, these unfortunates died of renal disease of "unknown etiology." Now, they survive with the aid of the artificial kidney, and can demand restitution for the injuries they incurred. But physicians have still to find a way to provide objective proof of the lead etiology after renal function has ceased entirely. The answer may yet reside within the bones. Laboratories in Sweden, Australia, and the United States (including my own) are vigorously exploring the possibility that bone lead content determined externally by X-ray induced X-ray fluorescence (XRF) can be used to measure body lead stores. If this approach is both accurate and safe, large-scale screening will be feasible. Those at risk of overt or insidious lead poisoning may then be identified and protected. Whether XRF will permit the prevention of lead poisoning in large populations will be determined by medical investigators over the next decade.

References
Index

References

1. Accum FC. *A Treatise on Adulterations of Food, and Culinary Poisons* . . . Philadelphia: Ab'm Small, 1820.
2. Ackerman A, Cronin E, Rodman D, Horan K, Hammond K, Aldaz L, Kellner R, Ouimette D, Dunn W, Fannin SL, Martinez A, Clin J. Lead poisoning from lead tetroxide used as a folk remedy—Colorado. *MMWR.* 1982; 30:646–47.
3. Acra A. Lead-glazed pottery: a potential health hazard in the Middle East. *Lancet.* 1981; ii:433–34.
4. Adams F. *The Genuine Works of Hippocrates.* London: Sydenham Society, 1849.
5. Aegineta P. *The Seven Books of Paulus Aegineta.* Translated by F Adams. London: Sydenham Society, 1844.
6. Agricola G. *De Re Metallica. 1556.* 1st ed. 1555. Translated by HC Hoover, LH Hoover. New York: Dover Publications, 1950.
7. ———. *De Natura Fossilium (Textbook of Mineralogy).* Translated by Bandy and Bandy. New York: Geological Society of America, 1955.
8. Aiello G. Ulteriori dati clinici ed istologici nelle nefropatie saturnine e nelle sclerosi renali non saturnine. *Med Lav.* 1931; 22:145–64.
9. Albahary C, Richet G, Guillaume J, Morel-Maroger L. Le rein dans le saturnisme professionnel. *Arch Mal Prof Med Trav Secur Soc.* 1965; 26:5–19.
10. Albahary C, Truhaut R, Boudene C, Desoille H. Le dépistage de l'imprégnation saturnine par un test de mobilisation du plomb. *La Presse Med.* 1961; 69:2121–23.
11. Alcock SK. The uncertainty of post-mortem evidence in suspected lead poisoning. *Br J Med.* 1905; 1:1371–73.
12. Alcock T. *The Endemial Colic of Devon, Not Caused By a Solution of Lead in the Cyder.* Plymouth: R Weatherby, 1769.
13. Alderson J. On the effects of lead upon the system. *Lancet.* 1852; ii:73–75/95–98.
14. Alessio L, Castoldi MR, Monelli O, Toffoletto F, Zochetti C. Indicators of internal dose in current and past exposure to lead. *Int Arch Occup Environ Health.* 1979; 44:127–32.
15. Allen AC. Acute lobular (membrano-proliferative) glomerulonephritis with hyperuricemia and obstructive uric acid nephropathy. *Am J Clin Pathol.* 1976; 65:109–20.
16. Allen BR, Hunter JAA, Beattie AD, Moore MR. Lead poisoning and blistering of the skin. *Scot Med J.* 1974; 19:3–6.

17. Angell ME, Relman AS, Robbins SL. Active chronic nephritis without evidence of bacterial infection. *N Engl J Med.* 1968; 278:1303–8.
18. Arnaud G. *A Dissertation of the Use of Goulard's Original Extract of Saturn, or Lead.* London, 1774.
19. Ask-Upmark E. Gout and the pathogenesis of its attacks. *Acta Med Scand.* 1967; 181:163–71.
20. Aslam M, Darig SS, Healy MA. Heavy metals in some Asian medicines and cosmetics. *Publ Hlth, Lond.* 1979; 93:274–84.
21. Atkins W. *A Discourse Shewing the Nature of the Gout.* London: T Fabian, 1694.
22. Aub JC, Fairhall LT, Minot AS, Reznikoff P. Lead poisoning. *Medicine.* 1925; 4:1–250.
23 Aufderheide AC, Neisman FD, Wittmers LE, Rapp G. Lead in bone II. Skeletal-lead content as an indicator of lifetime lead ingestion and the social correlates in an archaelogical population. *Am J Phys Anthropol.* 1981; 55:285–91.
24 Aurelianus C. *Caelinus Aurelianus.* Translated by IE Drabkin. Chicago: Univ. Press, 1950.
25. Avicenna. *A Treatise on the Canon of Medicine of Avicenna . . .* Translated by OC Gruner. London: Luzac, 1930.
26. Aviv A, John E, Bernstein J, Goldsmith DI, Spitzer A. Lead intoxication during development: its late effects on kidney function and blood pressure. *Kidney Int.* 1980; 17:430–37.
27. Baez J. *The Joan Baez Songbook.* New York: Reyerson Music Publishers, 1964.
28. Baker EL, Goyer RA, Fowler BA, Khettry U, Bernard DB, Adler S, White R de V, Babayan R, Feldman RG. Occupational renal exposure, nephropathy and renal cancer. *Am J Industr Med.* 1980; 1:139–48.
29. Baker EL, Landrigan PJ, Barbour AG, Cox DH, Folland DS, Ligo RN, Throckmorton J. Occupational lead poisoning in the United States: clinical and biochemical findings related to blood lead levels. *Br J Ind Med.* 1979; 36:314–22.
30. Baker G. *An Essay Concerning the Cause of the Endemial Colic of Devonshire* (1767). Reprint. Baltimore: Delta Omega Soc, 1958.
31. ———. An inquiry concerning the cause of the endemial colic of Devonshire (1768). 3rd ed. *Med Tr, Lond.* 1785; 1:175–256.
32. ———. An examination of several means, by which the poison of lead may be supposed frequently to gain admittance into the human body, unobserved and unsuspected (1768). 3rd ed. *Med Tr, Lond.* 1785; 1:257–318.
33. ———. An attempt towards an historical account of that species of spasmodic colic, distinguished by the name of colic of Poitou (1768). 3rd ed. *Med Tr, Lond.* 1785; 1:319–63.
34. ———. An examination of the several causes to which the colic of Poitou has been attributed (1768). 3rd ed. *Med Tr, Lond.* 1785; 1:364–406.
35. ———. Farther observations on the poison of lead. 2nd ed. *Med Tr, Lond.* 1771; 2:419–70.

36. ———. Additional observations concerning the colic of Poitou. *Med Tr, Lond.* 1785; 3:407–47.

37. Baker MD, Johnston JR, Maclatchy AE, Bezuidenhout BN. The relationship of serum uric acid to subclinical blood lead. *Rheum Rehab.* 1981; 20: 208–10.

38. Baldi G, Sbertoli C. Evoluzione delle alterazioni renali che possono condurre al rene grinzo saturnino: un caso dimostrativo. *Med Lav.* 1957; 48: 533–38.

39. Ball GV. Two epidemics of gout. *Bull Hist Med.* 1971; 45:401–8.

40. ———. Lead poisoning. In: Medical grand rounds from the University of Alabama Medical Center. *South Med J.* 1972; 65:278–87.

41. Ball GV, Sorenson, LB. Pathogenesis of hyperuricemia in saturnine gout. *N Engl J Med.* 1969; 280:1199–1202.

42. Barlow KA, Beilin LJ. Renal disease in primary gout. *Q J Med.* 1968; 37:79–98.

43. Barrough P. *Method of Physic.* 7th ed. London: Richard Field, 1590.

44. Barry PSI. A comparison of concentrations of lead in human tissues. *Br J Ind Med.* 1975; 32:119–39.

45. Basham WR. *Renal Diseases: A Clinical Guide to their Diagnosis and Treatment.* Philadelphia: Henry C Lea, 1870.

46. Batuman V, Landy E, Maesaka JK, Wedeen RP. Contribution of lead to hypertension with renal impairment. *N Engl J Med.* 1983; 309:17–21.

47. Batuman V, Maesaka JK, Haddad B, Tepper E, Landy E, Wedeen, RP. The role of lead in gout nephropathy. *N Engl J Med.* 1981; 304:520–23.

48. Bauer W. The diagnosis of gout. *N Engl J Med.* 1943; 229:583–90.

49. Beattie AD, Briggs JD, Canavan JSF, Dayle D, Mullin PJ, Watson AA. Acute lead poisoning: five cases resulting from self-injection of lead and opium. *Q J Med.* 1975; 174:275–84.

50. Beck LC. *Adulterations of Various substances Used in Medicine and the Arts.* New York: Samuel S and William Wood, 1846.

51. Beck TR. *Elements of Medical Jurisprudence.* Albany: Wester and Skinner, 1823.

52. Beevers DG, Cruickshank JK, Yeoman WB, Carter GF, Goldberg A, Moore MR. Blood-lead and cadmium in human hypertension. *J. Environ Pathol Toxicol.* 1980; 3:251–60.

53. Beevers DG, Erskine E, Robertson M, Beattie AD, Campbell BC, Goldberg A, Moore MR, Hawthorne VM. Blood-lead and hypertension. *Lancet.* 1976; ii:1–3.

54. Begbie JW. Observations in clinical medicine: lead impregnation and its connexion with gout and rheumatism. *Edinb Med J.* 1862; 8:125–32.

55. Begin ME. *Wine in the Different Forms of Anemia and Atonic Gout.* Paris: JB Baillière, 1877.

56. Beissat AAGA. *Etude sur l'albuminurie dans le saturnisme.* Dijon: Imprimerie Darantiere, 1894.

57. Belknap EL. Clinical studies on lead absorption in the human. III. Blood pressure observations. *J Ind Hyg Toxicol.* 1936; 18:380–90.

58. Bell J. *An Enquiry into the Causes which Produce and the Means of Preventing Diseases among British Officers, Soldiers and Others in the West-Indies.* London: J Murray, 1791.

59. Bell WB, Williams WR, Cunningham L. The toxic effects of lead administered intravenously. *Lancet.* 1925; ii:793–800.

60. Bence-Jones H. *On Gravel, Calculus & Gout: Chiefly an Application of Professor Liebig's Physiology to the Prevention and Cure of these Diseases.* London: Taylor, Walton, 1842.

61. Bence-Jones H. *Lectures on some of the Applications of Chemistry to Mechanics and Therapeutics.* London: John Churchill and Sons, 1867.

62. Berger L, Yü TF. Renal function in gout. IV. An analysis of 524 gouty subjects including long-term follow-up studies. *Am J Med.* 1975; 59:605–13.

63. Berkenhout J. *Doctor Cadogen's Dissertation on the Gout and All other Chronic Diseases Examined and Refuted.* London: S Bladon, 1772.

64. Bertel O, Buhler FR, Ott J. Lead-induced hypertension: blunted beta-adrenoceptor-mediated functions. *Brit Med J.* 1978; 1:551.

65. Betts PR, Astley R, Raine D. Lead intoxication in children in Birmingham. *Brit Med J.* 1973; 1:402–6.

66. Bidwell EH. Lead poisoning from an unusual source. *Med News.* 1887; 1:97.

67. Biggs N. *Mataeotechnia Medicinae Praxews. The Vanity of the Craft of Physic . . .* London: Giles Calvert, 1651.

68. Bird TD, Wallace DM, Labbe RF. The porphyria, plumbism, pottery puzzle. *JAMA.* 1982; 247:813–14.

69. Biringuccio V. *The Pirotechnia of Vanoccio Biringuccio.* Cambridge: MIT Press, 1966.

70. Blackall J. *Observations on the Nature and Cure of Dropsies, and Particularly on the Presence of the Coagulable Part of Blood in Dropsical Urine.* 4th ed. London: Longman, Hurst, Rees, Orme, Brown, Green, 1824.

71. Blackfan KD. Lead poisoning in children with especial reference to lead as a cause of convulsions. *Am J Med Sci.* 1917; 153:877–87.

72. Blackmore R. *Discourses On the Gout, Rheumatism and the King's Evil . . .* London: J Pemberton, 1726.

73. Bluestone R, Waisman J, Klinenberg JR. The gouty kidney. *Sem Arthritis Rheum.* 1977; 7:97–112.

74. Blumberg BS. Heredity of gout and hyperuricemia. *Arthritis Rheum.* 1965; 8:627–34.

75. Blyth AW. *Poisons: Their Effects and Detection.* New York: William Wood, 1885.

76. Board of the Assistant Alderman of the City of New York. *Report and Resolution on Zinc Paints.* New York: McSpedon and Baker, 1852.

77. Boerhaave H. *Boerhaave's Aphorisms: Concerning the Knowledge and Cure of Diseases.* Translated by J Delacoste. London: B Cousse, W Innys, 1715.

78. Bonet T. *A Guide to the Practical Physician . . .* London: Thomas Flesher, 1684.

79. Bordeu T. Sur le traitement de la colique métallique a l'Hôpital de la Charité de Paris, pour servir a l'histoire de la colique vulgairement nommée colique de Poitu. *J de Med Chir et Pharmacol.* 1762; 16:11–32.

80. Boss GR, Seegmiller JE. Hyperuricemia and gout: classification, complications, and management. *N Engl J Med.* 1979; 300:1459–68.

81. Bostocke R (RB). *The Differences Betwene the Auncient Physicke, first taught by the godly forefathers, consisting in unitie peace and concord: and the latter Physicke proceeding from Idolaters, Ethnickes, and Heathen: as Gallen, and such other consisting in dualitie, discorde, and contrarietie.* London: Robert Walley, 1585.

82. Boulin R, Violle PL. A propos d'un cas de goutte saturnine. *Rev Med.* 1938; 5:286–94.

83. Bouvart P. *Examen d'un livre qui a pour titre T Tronchin . . . de colica pictonum par un médicin de Paris.* Unpublished translation by M. Clements. Geneva, 1758.

84. ———. *Examen d'un livre qui a pour titre T Tronchin . . . de colica pictonum par un médicin de Paris.* 2nd ed. Geneva, 1767.

85. Bowie EA, North JDK. Allopurinol in treatment of patients with gout and chronic renal failure. *NZ Med J.* 1967; 66:606–11.

86. Bowman W. On the structure and use of Malpighian bodies of the kidney, with observations on the circulation through that gland. *Philosoph Tr Roy Soc, Lond.* 1842; 4:57–80.

87. Brahams D. Wasting medical expert's time. *Lancet.* 1982; ii:995.

88. Brande WT. An account of some changes from disease in the composition of human urine. *Tr Soc Improve Med Chir Knowledge.* 1807; 3:187–93.

89. Breckenridge A. Hypertension and hyperuricaemia. *Lancet.* 1966; i:15–18.

90. Brian T. *The Pisse-Prophet or Certain Pisse-Pot Lectures.* London: E.P., 1637.

91. Brieger H, Reiders F. Chronic lead and mercury poisoning: contemporary views on ancient occupational diseases. *J Chronic Dis.* 1959; 9:177–84.

92. Bright R. *Reports of Medical Cases, Selected with a View of Illustrating the Symptoms and Cure of Diseases by a Reference to Morbid Anatomy.* London: Longman, Rees, Orme, Brown, Green, 1827.

93. ———. Cases and observations, illustrative of renal disease accompanied with the secretion of albuminous urine. *Guy's Hosp Rep, Lond.* 1836; 1:338–400.

94. Briney WG, Ogden D, Bartholomew B, Smyth CJ. The influence of allopurinol on renal function in gout. *Arthritis Rheum.* 1975; 18:877–81.

95. Brochner-Mortensen K. 100 gouty patients. *Acta Med Scand.* 1941; 106:81–107.

96. Brogsitter AM, Wodarz H. Nierenveränderungen bei Bleivergiftung und Gicht. *Dtsch Arch Klin Med.* 1922; 139:129–42.

97. ———. *Histopathologie der Gelenk-Gicht.* Liepzig: Vogel, 1927.

98. Brouardel P. *Les intoxications.* Paris: JB Baillière, 1904.

99. Brown J. *The Elements of Medicine of John Brown, MD.* Translated by T Beddoes. Portsmouth: William Daniel Treadwell, 1803.

100. Brown J, Mallory GK. Renal changes in gout. *N Engl J Med.* 1950; 243:325–29.

101. Brown SS, ed. *Clinical Chemistry and Toxicology of Metals.* Elsevir: North Holland Biomed Pub Co, 1977.

102. Brunner JC. De experimento circa novam litargyrii. Unpublished transla-

tion by M. Sollenberger. *Miscellanea Curiosa, sive Ephemeridum Medico-Physicarum Germanicarum Curiosarum, Annus Secundus, Anni scilicet DCLXXI.* Frankfurt, 1688, pp. 193–96.

103. Buchan W. *Domestic Medicine . . .* Philadelphia: R Aitken, 1772.

104. ―――. *Domestic Medicine . . .* 3rd ed. London: W Strahan, T Cadell, 1774.

105. Buckingius JJ. *Consulatio Medico-Practica Proponens Aegrotum Arthritico-Nephriticum.* Unpublished translation by M. Sollenberger. Jena: Samuel Krebs, 1675.

106. Burton R. *Anatomy of Melancholy.* 8th ed. London: Peter Parker, 1676.

107. Bush JE. Case of pulmonary disease threatening phthisis, relieved by the supervention of colica pictonum, in consequence of drinking cider impregnated with lead. *West J Med Phys Sci.* 1831; 4:489–92.

108. Byrn ML. *Detection and Fraud and Protection of Health. A Treatise on the Adulteration of Food and Drink . . .* Philadelphia: Lippincott, Grambo, 1852.

109. Bywaters EGL. Gout in the time and person of George IV: a case history. *Ann Rheum Dis.* 1962; 21:325–38.

110. Cadogen W. *A Dissertation on the Gout . . .* 10th ed. London: Henry Knox, 1772.

111. Cadwalader T. *An Essay on the West-India Dry-Gripes . . .* Philadelphia: Franklin, 1745.

112. Caffey J. Lead poisoning associated with active rickets—report of a case with absence of lead lines in the skeleton. *Am J Dis Child.* 1938; 55: 798–806.

113. Campbell BC, Beattie AD, Elliott HL, Goldberg A, Moore MR, Beevers DG, Tree M. Occupational lead exposure and renin release. *Arch Environ Health.* 1979; 34:439–43.

114. Campbell BC, Beattie AD, Moore MR, Goldberg A, Reid AG. Renal insufficiency associated with excessive lead exposure. *Br Med J.* 1977; 1: 482–85.

115. Campbell BC, Elliott HL, Meredith PA. Lead exposure and renal failure: does renal insufficiency influence lead kinetics? *Toxicol Letters.* 1981; 9:121–24.

116. Campbell BC, Moore MR, Goldberg A. Subclinical lead exposure: a possible cause of gout. *Br Med J* 1978; 2:1403.

117. Cannon PJ, Stasm WB, Demartini FE, Sommers SC, Laragh JH. Hyperuricemia in primary and renal hypertension. *N Engl J Med.* 1966; 275:457–64.

118. Cantarow A, Trumper M. *Lead Poisoning.* Baltimore: Williams and Wilkins, 1944.

119. Carpenter WB. *On the Use and Abuse of Alcoholic Liquors in Health and Disease.* Boston: W Crosby, HP Nichols, 1851.

120. Carter W. *A Free and Candid Examination of Dr Cadogen's Dissertation on the Gout . . .* Canterbury: Simmons and Kirkby, 1771.

121. Castelnau, de, H. Observations et réflexions sur la goutte et le rhumatisme, et specialement sur quelques accidents graves qui peuvent se manifester dans le cours de ces deux affections. *Arch Gen de Med, Par.* 1843; 3: 285–314.

122. Caverhill J. *A Treatise On the Cause and Cure of the Gout*. London: G Scott, 1769.

123. Chapman EM. Observations on the effect of paint on the kidneys with particular reference to the role of turpentine. *J Ind Hyg Toxicol*. 1941; 23: 277–89.

124. Chapman N. *Lectures on the More Important Eruptive Fevers, Hemorrhages and Dropsies and on Gout and Rheumatism*. Philadelphia: Lea and Blanchard, 1844.

125. Charcot J-M. *Etudes pour servir à l'historie de l'affection décrite sous les noms de goutte asthénique primitive nodosités des jointures, rhumatisme articulaire chronique (forme primitive) etc*. Paris: Rignoux, 1853.

126. ⸺. L'intoxication saturnine exerce-t-elle une influence sur le développement de la goutte? *Gaz Hebd de Med, Par*. 1863; 10:434–39.

127. ⸺. *Leçons sur les maladies vieillards et les maladies chroniques*. 1st ed. 1864. Paris: Adrien Delahaye, 1868.

128. ⸺. *Lectures on Bright's Disease of the Kidneys*. Translated by HB Millard. New York: William Wood, 1879.

129. ⸺. *Clinical Lectures on Senile and Chronic Diseases*. Translated by WS Tuke. London: New Sydenham Society, 1881.

130. ⸺. *Clinical Lectures on the Diseases of Old age*. Translated by L H Hunt. New York: William Wood, 1881.

131. Charcot J-M, Cornil V. Contributions a l'étude des altérations anatomiques de la goutte, et spécialement du rein chez les goutteux. *Compt Rend Soc de Biol, Par*. 1864; 15:139–63.

132. Charcot J-M, Gombault. Note relative a l'étude anatomique de la néphrite saturnine expérimentale. *Arch Physiol*. 1881; 8:126–54.

133. Charleton R. *Three Tracts on Bath waters*. Bath: R Crattwell for W Taylor, 1774.

134. Chevallier A. Note sur le plomb et sur les accidents déterminés par ce métal, ses oxides et ses composés. *Ann d'Hyg, Par*. 1842; 28:224–27.

135. Cheyne G. *An Essay of the True Nature and Due Method of Treating the Gout*. 9th ed. London: G Strahan, 1738.

136. ⸺. *An Essay on Regimen . . .* London: C Rivington, J Leake, 1740.

137. Children's Employment Commission (1862). *First Report of the Commissioner's on the Employment of Children and Young Persons in Trades and Manufactures with an Appendix*. Facsimile. Shannon: Irish Univ. Press, 1968.

138. Childs SJR. Sir George Baker and the dry belly-ache. *Bull Hist Med*. 1970; 44:213–40.

139. Chisolm JJ. Aminoaciduria as a manifestation of renal tubular injury in lead intoxication and as a comparison wth patterns of aminoaciduria seen in other diseases. *J Pediatr*. 1962; 60:1–17.

140. ⸺. Chelation therapy in children with subclinical plumbism. *Ped*. 1974; 53:441–43.

141. Chisolm JJ, Harrison HC, Eberlern WR, Harrison HE. Aminoaciduria, hypophosphatemia and rickets in lead poisoning. *Am J Dis Child*. 1955; 89: 159–68.

142. Chmielnicka J, Komsta-Szumanska E, Szymanska JA. Arginase and kallikrein activities as biochemical indices of occupational exposure to lead. *Br J Ind Med.* 1981; 38:175–78.

143. Christison R. Observations on the variety of dropsy which depends on diseased kidney. *Edinb Med Surg J.* 1829; 32:262–91.

144. ———. *Granular Degeneration of the Kidneys, and Its Connection with Dropsy, Inflammation, and Other Diseases.* Philadelphia: A Waldie, 1839.

145. ———. *A Treatise on Poisons in Relation to Medical Jurisprudence, Physiology and the Practice of Physic.* 4th ed. Edinburgh: Adam and Charles Black, 1845.

146. Citois F. *De Novoet Populari Colico Bilioso Dolore Diatriba.* Unpublished translation by M. Sollenberger. Paris: Montpellier, 1639.

147. Cobbett W. *Porcupine's Gazette.* 1800; 779:52–62.

148. Cogan T. *The Haven of Health.* London: Henrie Middleton for William Morton, 1584.

149. Cohnheim J. *Lectures on General Pathology.* Translated by AB McKee. London: New Sydenham Society, 1890.

150. Colbatch J. *A Treatise of the Gout. . .* London: Daniel Brown, Roger Clavel, 1697.

151. Cole JF. Blood lead. *J Occup Med.* 1975; 17:348.

152. Colton RS. Ward LF, Maher FT. Occult renal impairment in gouty and hyperuricemic individuals. *Am J Med Sci.* 1966; 252:575–79.

153. Colwells, Shaw, Willard. *Manufacture of Willard and Shaw's Patent Tin Lined Lead Pipes.* New York: Slater and Riley, 1865.

154. Committee. *The Case of the County of Devon, with Respect to the Consequences of the New Excise Duty on Cyder and Perry.* London: W Johnston, B Thorn, 1763.

155. Coombs FS, Pecora LJ, Thorogood E, Consolazio NV, Talbott JH. Renal function in patients with gout. *J Clin Invest.* 1940; 19:525–35.

156. Cooper WC, Gaffey WR. Mortality of lead workers. *J Occup Med.* 1975; 17:100–107.

157. Copeman WSC. *A Short History of the Gout and the Rheumatic Diseases.* Berkeley: Univ. of Calif. Press, 1964.

158. Copeman WSC, Winder M. The first medical monograph on the gout. On whether it is possible to cure the gout or no. *Med Hist.* 1969; 13:288–93.

159. Cornil V. *Des Différences Espèces de Néphrites.* Thèse présentée et soutenue a la Faculté de Médicine. Paris: Germer Baillière, 1869.

160. Corson JW. On the effects of lead on the heart. *NY J Med.* 1856; 16:234–55.

161. Cotugno D. *A Treatise on the Nervous Sciatica, or, Nervous Hip Gout.* Translated by H Crantz. London: J Wilkie, 1775.

162. ———. His description of the cerebrospinal fluid, with a translation of part of his *De Ischiade Nervosa Commentarius* (1764), and a bibliography of his important works. Translated by HR Viets. *Bull Hist Med.* 1935; 3:701–38.

163. Cowen DL. *Medicine and Health in New Jersey: A History.* New Jersey Historical Series. Vol 16. Princeton: D Van Nostrand, 1964.

164. Cramer K, Dahlberg L. Incidence of hypertension among lead workers: a follow-up study based on regular control over 20 years. *Brit J Ind Med.* 1966; 23:101−4.

165. Cramer K, Goyer RA, Jagenburg R, Marion H. Renal ultrastructure, renal function, and parameters of lead toxicity in workers with different periods of lead exposure. *Br J Ind Med.* 1974; 31:113−27.

166. Crampton J. Clinical report on dropsies. *King and Queens Coll Phys Tr.* 1818; 2:140−274.

167. Crawford H. A recent acute case of lead poisoning in Brisbane and associated with haematoporphyrinuria. *Med J Aust.* 1933:589.

168. Crepet M, Chiesura P, Gobbato F. Comportamemto della funzione renale nella intossicazione professionale da piombo. *Folia Med.* 1953; 36:181−96.

169. Crosby WH. Lead contaminated health food: the tip of the iceberg. *JAMA.* 1977; 238:1544.

170. Crutcher JC. Clinical manifestations and therapy of acute lead intoxication due to the ingestion of illicitly distilled alcohol. *Ann Intern Med.* 1963; 59:707−15.

171. Cullen TF. Colica Pictonum. report of the standing committee. *Tr Med Soc NJ.* 1869:131−33.

172. Cullen W. *First Lines of the Practice of Physic . . .* Translated by J Rotheram. New York: Samuel Cambell, 1793.

173. Culpeper N. *Pharmacopoeia Londinensis: Or the London Dispensory.* 6th ed. London: Peter Cole, 1653.

174. Curio J, Crellius J. *De Conservanda Bona Valetudine Opusculum Scholae Salernitanae . . .* Franc. Apud Chr. Egen. 1551.

175. Currie W. *An Historical Account of the Climates and Diseases of the United States of America . . .* Philadelphia: T Dobson, 1792. Reprint. New York: Arno Press, 1972.

176. Dagg JH, Goldberg A, Lockhead A, Smith JA. The relationship of lead poisoning to acute intermittent porphyria. *Q J Med.* 1965; 34:163−75.

177. Danilovic V. Chronic nephritis due to ingestion of lead-contaminated flour. *Brit J Med.* 1958; 1:27−28.

178. Danjoy L. De l'albuminurie dans l'encéphalopathie et l'amaurose saturnines. *Arch Gen de Med, Par.* 1864; 1:402−23.

179. Danmoniensis. *An Answer to Dr. Baker's Essay Concerning the Cause of the Endemial Colic of Devonshire, wherein the Cyder of that County is Exculpated from the Accusation Brought Against it by that Gentleman.* Exeter: R Trewman, 1767.

180. Darwin C. *Experiments Establishing a Criterion between Mucilaginous and Purulent Matter and An Account of the Retrograde Motions of the Absorbent Vessels of Animal Bodies in some Diseases.* Edinburg: E Darwin, 1780.

181. Darwin E. *Zoonomia: or, the Laws of Organic Life.* London: Thomas J Johnson, 1796.

182. ———. *The Letters of Erasmus Darwin.* King-Hele D, ed. Cambridge: At the Univ. Press, 1981.

183. Day RS, Eales L. Porphyrins in chronic renal failure. *Nephron.* 1980; 26: 90–95.

184. Day RS, Eales L, Disler PB. Porphyrias and the kidney. *Nephron.* 1981; 28:261–67.

185. Day RS, Eales L, Meissner D. Coexistent variegate porphyria and porphyria cutanea tarda. *N Engl J Med.* 1982; 307:37–41.

186. Debus GA. *The English Paracelsians.* New York: Franklin Watts, 1965.

187. Demartini FE. Hyperuricemia induced by drugs. *Arthritis Rheum.* 1965; 8:823–27.

188. Dickens C. *The Uncommercial Traveller.* New York: Books Inc, 1868.

189. Dickinson WH. *On the Pathology and Treatment of Albuminuria.* London: Longmans, Green, 1868.

190. ———. *A Treatise on Albuminuria.* 2nd ed. New York: William Wood, 1881.

191. Dingwall-Fordyce I, Lane RE. A follow-up of lead workers. *Br J Ind Med.* 1963; 20:313–15.

192. Dioscorides. *The Greek Herbal of Dioscorides.* Translated by J Goodyer, 1655. Gunther RT, ed. New York: Hafner Pub Co, 1959.

193. Dobbs BJT. *The Foundations of Newton's Alchemy or "The Hunting of the Greene Lyon".* Cambridge: Cambridge Univ. Press, 1975.

194. Dock W., trans. De ischiade nervosa commentarius, 1765–1775, by Domenico Cotugno. *Ann Med Hist.* 1922; 4:287–96.

195. Donald GF, Hunter GA, Roman W, Taylor AE. Current concepts of cutaneous porphyria and its treatment with particular reference to the use of sodium calcium edetate. *Br J Dermatol.* 1970; 82:70–75.

196. Donne J. The canonization. In: Hebel JW, Hudson HH, eds. *Poetry of the English Renaissance, 1509–1660.* New York: Appleton-Century-Crofts, 1929.

197. Doss A., ed. *Porphyrins in Human Disease.* New York: S Karger, 1976.

198. ———. *Diagnosis and Therapy of Porphyrias and Lead Intoxication.* New York: Springer-Verlag, 1978.

199. Drake D. *A Systematic Treatise . . . on the Principal Diseases of the Interior Valley of North America . . .* Cincinnati: Winthrop B Smith, 1850.

200. Drake R. *An Essay on the Nature and Manner of Treating the Gout.* London: Drake, 1751.

201. ———. *A Candid and Impartial Account of the Very Great Probability that there is Discovered a Specific in the Gout . . .* London, 1771.

202. Drash GA. Lead burden in prehistorical, historical and modern human bones. *Science Total Environ.* 1982; 24:199–231.

203. Dressen WC. Health of lead exposed storage battery workers. *J Ind Hyg Toxicol.* 1943; 25:60–70.

204. Duckworth D. *A Treatise on Gout.* Philadelphia: SM Blakiston, 1889.

205. Dufour M, Choisy H, Morice MT. Lead glazed pottery in France. *Lancet.* 1972; 1:1008.

206. Dugas LA. Cases of colica pictonum. *South Med Surg J.* 1837; 1:402–3.

207. Duncan H, Dixon ASJ. Gout, familial hyperuricaemia and renal disease. *Q J Med.* 1960; 29:127–35.

208. Duncan H, Wakim KG. Renal lesions resulting from induced hyperuricemia in animals. *Proc Mayo Clin.* 1963; 38:411–21.

209. Dunn JP, Brooks GW, Mausner J, Rodnan GP, Cobb S. Social class gradient of serum uric acid levels in males. *JAMA.* 1963; 185:431–36.

210. Dunn JS, Polson CJ. Experimental uric acid nephritis. *J Pathol Bacteriol.* 1926; 29:337–52.

211. Eales L, Dowdle EB. Clinical aspects of importance in the porphyrias. *Brit J Clin Pract.* 1968; 22:505–15.

212. Ebell GU. Ueber die Bleyglasur unserer Töpferwaare. Hannover: TE Lamminger, 1794.

213. Editor. Advertisement. *Med Tr, Lond.* 1768:5–9.

214. ———. Nephropathy in chronic lead poisoning. *JAMA.* 1966; 197:722.

215. ———. Acute renal failure in lead poisoning. *Lancet.* 1978; ii:140.

216. ———. Immunogenetics and essential hypertension. *Lancet.* 1978; ii:409–10.

217. ———. Sir Isaac Newton and his madness of 1692–1695. *Lancet.* 1980; i:529–30.

218. ———. Alcoholic heart disease. *Lancet.* 1980; i:961–62.

219. ———. Hypertension and uric acid. *Lancet.* 1981; i:365–66.

220. ———. Surveillance of childhood lead poisoning—United States. *MMWR.* 1982; 31:118–19.

221. Ehrlich GE, Chokatos J. Saturnine gout. *Arch Intern Med.* 1966; 118:572–74.

222. Eisinger J. Lead and man. *Trends Biochem Sci.* 1977; 2:N147–50.

223. ———. Leaded wine: Eberhard Gockel and the colica Pictonum. *Medical History.* 1982; 26:279–302.

224. Ellenbog U. *Von den gifftigen besen Tempffen und Reuchen.* Munich: Der Müchner Drucke, 1927.

225. ———. On the poisonous evil vapours and fumes of metals such as silver, quicksilver, lead and others . . . Translated by C Barnard. *Lancet.* 1932; i:270–71.

226. Ellwanger GH. *Meditations on Gout with a Consideration of its Cure Through the Use of Wine.* Cambridge: Univ. Press, John Wilson and Son, 1897.

227. Emmerson BT. Chronic lead nephropathy: the diagnostic use of calcium EDTA and the association with gout. *Aust Ann Med.* 1963; 12:310–24.

228. ———. The renal excretion of urate in chronic lead nephropathy. *Aust Ann Med.* 1965; 14:295–303.

229. ———. The clinical differentiation of lead gout from primary gout. *Arthritis Rheum.* 1968; 11:623–34.

230. ———. Chronic lead nephropathy. *Kidney Int.* 1973; 4:1–5.

231. ———. Gout, uric acid and renal disease. *Med J Aust.* 1976; 1:403–5.

232. ———. Atherosclerosis and urate metabolism. *Aust NZ J Med.* 1979; 9:451–54.

233. ———. The kidney and gout. In: Hamburger J, Crosnier J, Grunfeld JP, eds. *Nephrology.* New York: John Wiley and Sons, 1979.

234. ———. Uricosuric diuretics. *Kidney Int.* 1980; 18:677–85.

235. Emmerson BT, Leckey DS. The lead content of bone in subjects without recognized past lead exposure and in patients with renal disease. *Aust Ann Med.* 1963; 12:139–42.

236. Emmerson BT, Mirosch W, Douglas JB. The relative contributions of tubular reabsorption and secretion to urate secretion in lead nephropathy. *Aust NZ J Med.* 1971; 4:353–61.

237. Emmerson BT, Row PG. An evaluation of the pathogenesis of the gouty kidney. *Kidney Int.* 1975; 8:65–71.

238. Emmerson BT, Thiele BR. Calcium versenate in the diagnosis of chronic lead nephropathy. *Med J Aust.* 1960; 1:243–48.

239. Environmental Protection Agency. *Lead-Air Quality Criteria Document.* Forthcoming.

240. Ernhart CB. Lead levels and confounding variables. *Am J Psychiatry.* 1982; 11:1524.

241. Eshner AA. A case of albuminuria and oxaluria presumably of plumbic origin. *Phil Polyclinic.* 1895; 4:294–95.

242. Eskew AE, Crutcher JC, Zimmerman SL, Johnston GW, Butz WC. Lead poisoning resulting from illicit alcohol consumption. *J Forensic Sci.* 1961; 6:337–50.

243. Espinasse N. *Robert Hooke.* Berkeley: Univ. of Calif. Press, 1962.

244. Evans DJ, Jones AE. The development of statutory safeguards against pneumoconiosis and lead poisoning in the North Staffordshire pottery industry. *Ann Occup Hyg.* 1974; 17:1–14.

245. Every RR. Bovine lead poisoning from forage contaminated by sandblasted paint. *J Am Vet Med Assoc.* 1981; 178:1277–78.

246. Ewart W. *The Nature, Causes, and Means of the Prevention of the Diseases incident to Lead Miners.* Carlisle: Jas Steel, 1846.

247. ———. *Gout and Goutiness: and Their Treatment.* London: Bailliere, Tindall and Cox, 1896.

248. Ewell J. *The Planter's and Mariner's Medical Companion . . .* Philadelphia: John Bioren, 1807.

249. Falconer W. *An Essay on the Bath Waters.* London: T Lowndes, 1770.

250. ———. *An Address To Doctor Cadogen Occasioned By His Dissertation On The Gout . . .* London: J Almon, 1771.

251. Felton JS. Man, medicine and work in America: an historical series. II. Lead, liquor and legislation. *J Occup Med.* 1965; 7:572–79.

252. ———. Man, medicine and work in America: an historical series. III. Benjamin Franklin and his awareness of lead poisoning. *J Occup Med.* 1967; 9:543–54.

253. ———. Man, medicine and work in America: an historical series. IV. Thomas Cadwalader MD: physician, Philadelphian and philanthropist. *J Occup Med.* 1969; 11:374–80.

254. Fenner ED. Special report on lead poisoning in New Orleans. *South Med Rep.* 1850; 2:247–80.

255. Fessel WJ. Renal outcomes of gout and hyperuricemia. *Am J Med.* 1979; 67:74–82.

256. ———. High uric acid as an indicator of cardiovascular disease. Independence from obesity. *Am J Med.* 1980; 68:401–4.

257. Fessel WJ, Siegelach AB, Johnson ES. Correlates and consequences of a symptomatic hyperuricemic. *Arch Dtsch Med.* 1973; 132:44–54.

258. Filby FA. *A History of Food Adulteration and Analysis.* London: George Allen & Unwin, 1934.

259. Findling JW, Beckstrom D, Rawsthorne L, Kozin F, Itskovitz H. Indomethacin-induced hyperkalemia in three patients with gouty arthritis. *JAMA.* 1980; 244:1127–28.

260. Fineberg SK, Altschul A. The nephropathy of gout. *Ann Intern Med.* 1956; 44:1182–94.

261. Fitz R. A note on the history of lead poisoning in Boston. *N Engl J Med.* 1934; 210:802–6.

262. Floyer J, Baynard E. *The History of Cold Bathing.* 6th ed. London: W Innys, R Mamby, 1732.

263. Forbes M. *A Treatise Upon Gravel and Upon Gout.* London: T Cadell, 1787.

264. ———. *A Treatise Upon Gravel and Gout.* London: T Cadell, 1793.

265. Fordyce G. *Elements of the Practice of Physic in Two Parts . . .* 5th ed. London: J Johnson, 1784.

266. Fothergill J. Observations on disorders to which painters in water colors are exposed. *Med Observational Inquires.* 1776; 5:394–405.

267. ———. *Cautions to the Heads of Families.* London, 1790.

268. Fothergill JM. *Gout in its Protean Aspects.* London: HK Lewis, 1883.

269. Fouts PJ, Page IH. The effect of chronic lead poisoning on arterial blood pressure in dogs. *Am Heart J.* 1942; 24:329–31.

270. Franklin B. *The Works of Benjamin Franklin.* Boston: Tappan and Whittemore, 1836.

271. ———. *Autobiography of Benjamin Franklin with Introduction and Notes.* New York: Macmillan, 1922.

272. Frazier PD, Seegmiller JE. Characterization of crystalline deposits in kidney tissue of patients with gout and with acute lymphocytic leukemia. *Arthritis Rheum.* 1966; 9:504.

273. Freedman LR. Pyelonephritis and urinary tract infection. In: Strauss MB, Welt LC, eds. *Diseases of the Kidney.* Boston: Little, Brown and Co, 1963.

274. Freeman, RB, Smith WM, Richardson JA, Hennelly PJ, Thurm RH, Urner C, Vaillancourt JA, Griep RJ, Bromfr L. Long term therapy for chronic bacteriuria in men. *Ann Intern Med.* 1975; 83:133–47.

275. Friend J. *The History of Physick . . .* 4th ed. London, 1744.

276. Fulton JF. Charles Darwin and the early use and history of digitalis. *Bull NY Acad Med.* 1934; 10:496–506.

277. Gadbury J. *Thesaurus Astrologie . . .* London: Thomas Passenger, 1674.

278. Gairdner W. *On Gout . . .* 2nd ed. London: John Churchill, 1851.

279. Galambos JT, Dowda FW. Lead poisoning and porphyria. *Am J Med.* 1959; 29:803–6.

280. Galambos JT, Peacock LB. The use of chelating agents in the treatment of acute porphyria. *Ann Intern Med.* 1959; 50:1056–61.

281. Gale NH, Stos-Gale ZA. Lead and silver in the ancient Aegean. *Scientific American.* 1981; 244:176–92.

282. ———. Bronze-age copper sources in the Mediterranean: a new approach. *Science.* 1982; 216:11–19.

283. Galle P, Morel-Maroger L. Les lésions rénales du saturnisme humain et expérimental. *Nephron.* 1965; 2:273–86.

284. Garrison FH. *An Introduction to the History of Medicine.* Philadelphia: WB Saunders, 1929.

285. Garrod AB. Observations on certain pathological conditions of the blood and urine in gout, rheumatism and Bright's disease. *Med Chir Tr, Lond.* 1847–48; 31:83–97.

286. ———. Second communication on the blood and effused fluids in gout, rheumatism and Brights' disease. *Med Chir Tr, Lond.* 1854; 37:49–61.

287. ———. Chronic gout. *Lancet.* 1856; i:97–98.

288. ———. Researches on gout. Part I. The urine in the different forms of gout. Part II. The influence of colchicum upon the urine. *Med Chir Tr, Lond.* 1858; 41:325–60.

289. ———. *The Nature and Treatment of Gout and Rheumatic Gout.* London: Walton and Maberly, 1859.

290. ———. Clinical remarks on a case of lead-poisoning. *Lancet.* 1870; ii:781–82.

291. ———. *A Treatise on Gout and Rheumatic Gout. (Rheumatoid Arthritis).* 3rd ed. London: Longmans, Green and Co, 1876.

292. ———. Eczema and albuminuria in relation to gout. *Tr Int Med Congress.* 1881; 7:99–202.

293. Garrod AE. On the occurrence and detection of haematoporphyria in the urine. *J Physiol.* 1892; 13:598–620.

294. ———. The Bradshaw lecture on the urinary pigments in their pathological aspects. *Lancet.* 1900; ii:1323–31.

295. Geach F. *Some Observations on Dr. Baker's Essay on the Endemial Colic of Devonshire.* London: R Baldwin, 1767.

296. ———. *A Reply to Dr. Saunders' Pamphlet, Relative to the Dispute Concerning the Devonshire Cider.* London: R Baldwin, 1768.

297. Geoffroy SF. *A Treatise of the Fossil, Vegetable and Animal Substances, that are Made Use of in Physick.* Translated by G Douglas. London: W Innys, R Manby, T Woodward, C Davis, 1736.

298. Geppert. Chronische Nephritis nach Bleivergiftung. *Dtsch Med Klin Wochenschr.* 1882; 8:241–42.

299. Gerhardt RE, Crecelius EA, Hudson JB. Trace element content of moonshine. *Arch Environ Health.* 1980; 35:332–34.

300. Gibson JL. Plumbic ocular neuritis in Queensland children. *Br J Med.* 1908; 2:1488–90.

301. Gibson JL, Love W, Hardie D, Bancroft P, Turner AJ. Notes on lead poisoning as observed among children in Brisbane. *Proc Intercolonial Med Congress: Aust.* 1892; 3:76–83.

302. Gibson T. Gout and hyperlipidaemia. *Adv Exp Med Biol.* 1974; 41B:499–508.

303. Gibson T, Highton J, Potter C, Simmonds HA. Renal impairment and gout. *Ann Rheum Dis.* 1980; 39:417–23.

304. Gibson T, Simmonds HA, Potter C, Jeyarajah W, Highton J. Gout and renal function. *Eur J Rheumatol Inflamm.* 1978; 1:79–85.

305. Gibson T, Simmonds HA, Potter C, Rogers V. A controlled study of the effect of allopurinol treatment on renal function in gout. In: Rapado A, Watts RWE, De Bruyn CHMM, eds. *Purine Metabolism in Man III.* New York: Plenum Press, 1980.

306. Gilfillan SC. Lead poisoning and the fall of Rome. *J Occup Med.* 1965; 7:53–60.

307. Gobbato F, Chiesura P. La nefropatia da piombo. *Minerva nefrologica.* 1968; 15:12–24.

308. Gockel E. *Vini Acidi per Acetum Lithargyri, cum Maximo Bibentium Damno Dulcificatione.* Unpublished translation by M. Sollenberger. 1697.

309. Goettsch E, Mason H. Glycosuria in lead poisoning. *Am J Dis Child.* 1940; 59:119–28.

310. Goldberg A. Lead poisoning as a disorder of heme synthesis. *Sem Hematol.* 1968; 5:424–33.

311. Goldwater LJ. *History of Quicksilver.* Baltimore: York Press, 1972.

312. Gonick HC, Rubini ME, Gleason IO, Sommers SC. The renal lesion in gout. *Ann Intern Med.* 1965; 62:667–74.

313. Gonzalez JJ, Werk EE, Thrasher K, Behar R, Loadholt B. Renin aldosterone system and potassium levels in chronic lead intoxication. *South Med J.* 1979; 72:433–36.

314. Goodfellow SJ. *Lectures on the Diseases of the Kidney, Generally Known as "Brights Disease", and the Dropsy.* London: Robert Hardwicke, 1861.

315. Gough JW. *The Mines of Mendip.* Newton Abbot, Devon: David and Charles, 1967.

316. Goulard T. *A Treatise on the Effects of Various Preparations of Lead, Particularly of the Extract of Saturn: for Different Chirurgical Disorders.* Translated by G Arnaud. London: P Elmsly, 1775.

317. Goyer RA, Tsuchiya K, Leonard DL, Kahyo H. Aminoaciduria in Japanese workers in the lead and cadmium industries. *Am J Clin Pathol.* 1972; 57:635–42.

318. Goyer RA, Wilson MH. Lead-induced inclusion bodies. Results of ethylene-diaminetetraacetic acid treatment. *Lab Invest.* 1975; 32:149–56.

319. Graham W. *The Art of Making Wines from Fruits, Flowers, and Herbs, All the Native Growth of Great Britain.* 3rd ed. London: W Nicoll, c. 1766.

320. Graham W, Graham KM. Our gouty past. *Can M A J.* 1955; 73:485–93.

321. Grahame R, Scott JT. Clinical survey of 354 patients with gout. *Ann Rheum Dis.* 1970; 29:461–68.

322. Grandjean P. Lead in Danes: historical & toxicological studies. In: Coulston F, Korte F, eds. *Environmental Quality & Safety.* Suppl 2:6–75. New York: Academic Press, 1975.

323. ———. Lead retention in ancient Nubian and contemporary populations. *J Environ Pathol Toxicol.* 1979; 2:781–87.

324. Granick JL. Some biochemical and clinical aspects of lead intoxication. *Adv Clin Chem*. 1978; 20:287–339.

325. Grant W. *Some Observations on the Origin, Progress and Method of Treating the Atrabilious Temperament and Gout*. London: T Cadell, 1779.

326. Granville JM. The mental element in the etiology of gout. *Lancet*. 1881; i:574–75.

327. Green SA. *History of Medicine in Massachusetts*. Boston: A Williams and Co, 1881.

328. Green TE. Some unusual forms of lead poisoning. *Aust Med Gaz*. 1897; 16:483–84.

329. Greenbaum D, Ross JH, Steinberg VL. Renal biopsy in gout. *Br Med J*. 1961; 1:1502–4.

330. Greenfield I, Gray I. Lead poisoning. IX. The failure of lead poisoning to affect the heart and blood vessels. *Am Heart J*. 1950; 39:430–35.

331. Gregory JC. On diseased states of the kidney connected during life with albuminous urine; illustrated by cases. *Edinb Med Surg J*. 1831; 36:315–63.

332. Gresham GE. Hyperuricemia. *Arch Environ Health*. 1965; 11:863–70.

333. Grew N. *Musaeum Regalis Societatis . . .* London: Hugh Newman, 1694.

334. Griffith JQ, Linauer MA. The effect of chronic lead poisoning on arterial blood pressure in rats. *Am Heart J*. 1944; 28:295–97.

335. Grisler R, Finulli M. Utilità della tecnica semplificata della clearance dell'acido paraaminoippurico nello studio della nefropatie vascolari professionali. *Med Lav*. 1960; 51:376–80.

336. Gross SB, Pfitzer EA, Yeager DW, Kehoe RA. Lead in human tissues. *Toxicol Appl Pharmacol*. 1975; 32:638–51.

337. Gross SD. *Lives of Eminent American Physicians and Surgeons of the Nineteenth Century*. Philadelphia: Lindsay and Blakiston, 1861.

338. ———. Human oral and inhalation exposure to lead: summary of Kehoe balance experiments. *J Toxicol Environ Health*. 1981; 8:333–77.

339. Gudbrandsson T. Immunological changes in patients with previous malignant essential hypertension. *Lancet*. 1981; i:406–7.

340. Gull W. Clinical lecture on chronic Bright's disease, with contracted kidney. *Brit Med J*. 1872:673–74, 707–9.

341. Gull W, Sutton HG. On the pathology of the morbid state commonly called capillary fibrosis. *Brit Med J*. 1872:620–22.

342. Gutman AB. Primary and secondary gout. *Ann Intern Med*. 1953; 39:1062–76.

343. Hadenque A, Collin M. Etudes sur la taux de l'azotémie des ouvriers exposés du plomb. *Bull Soc Med Hyg du Travail*. 1951; 12:561–65.

344. Haen, de, A. *Dissertation on Colica Pictonum*. Unpublished translation by M Sollenberger. The Hague: Batavia, 1745.

345. Haig A. *Uric Acid as a Factor in the Causation of Disease . . .* 5th ed. London: J and A Churchill, 1900.

346. Hall A. The increasing use of lead as an abortifacient. *Brit Med J*. 1905; 1:582–87.

347. Halla JT, Ball G. Saturnine gout: a review of 42 patients. *Sem Arthritis Rheum.* 1982; 11:307–14.

348. Hamilton A. *Industrial Poisons in the United States.* New York: Macmillan, 1929.

349. ———. *Exploring the Dangerous Trades: The Autobiography of Alice Hamilton, MD.* Boston: Little, Brown and Co, 1943.

350. Hamilton J. *Observations on the Use and Abuse of Mercurial Medicines.* New York: E Bliss, E White, 1821.

351. Hamilton R. *Letters on the Cause and Treatment of the Gout . . .* 2nd ed. London: W Whittingham, 1808.

352. Hansen OE. Hyperuricemia, gout, and atherosclerosis. *Am Heart J.* 1966; 72:570–73.

353. Hardy J. *A Candid Examination of what has been Advanced as the Colic of Poitou and Devonshire, with Remarks on the Most Probable and Experiments Intended to Ascertain the True Causes of Gout.* Devonshire: J Hardy, 1778.

354. ———. *An Answer to the Letter Addressed by Francis Riolloy, Physician of Newbury to Dr Hardy, on the Hints Given Concerning the Origin of the Gout, in his Publication on the Colic of Devon.* London: T Cadell, 1780.

355. Harlan R. Observations on colica Pictonum, and other affections arising from the deleterious operation of lead on the system. *North Am Med Surg J.* 1828; 5:16–23.

356. Harrington J. *The School of Salernum . . .* Notes by F. R. Packard and F. H. Garrison. New York: Paul B Hoeber, 1920.

357. Harris LT. A clinical study of the frequency of lead, temperature and benzoin poisoning in four hundred painters. *Arch Intern Med.* 1918; 22:129–56.

358. Harrison JB. *Some Observations on the Contamination of Water by the Poison of Lead . . .* London: John Churchill, 1852.

359. Hartung EF. History of the use of colchicum and related medicaments on gout, with suggestions for further research. *Ann Rheum Dis.* 1954; 13:190–200.

360. Hassall AH. *Food and its Adulterations. Comprising the Analytical Sanitary Commission of "The Lancet" for the Years 1851–1855 Inclusive.* London: Longman, Brown, Green and Longmans, 1855.

361. Havelda CJ, Sohi GS, Richardson CE. Evaluation of lead, zinc and copper excretion in chronic moonshine drinkers. *South Med J.* 1980; 73:710–15.

362. Hayman JM. Malpighi's "Concerning the Structure of the Kidneys": a translation and introduction. *Ann Med Hist.* 1925; 7:242–63.

363. Healey LA. Port wine and the gout. *Arthritis Rheum.* 1975; 18:659–62.

364. Heberden W. *Commentaries on the History and Cure of Diseases* (1802). New York: Hafner Publishing Co, 1962.

365. Henderson. 128th Meeting of Medical Society of Queensland. *Aust Med Gaz.* 1897; 16:519.

366. Henderson DA. A follow-up of cases of plumbism in children. *Aust Ann Med.* 1954; 3:219.

367. ———. Chronic nephritis in Queensland. *Aust Ann Med.* 1955; 4:163–.

368. ———. The aetiology of chronic nephritis in Queensland. *Med J Aust.* 1958; 1:377–86.

369. Henderson DA, Inglis JA. The lead content of bone in chronic Brights disease. *Aust Ann Med.* 1957; 6:145–54.

370. Heptinstall RH. *Pathology of the Kidney.* 2nd ed, Boston: Little, Brown and Co, 1974.

371. ———. Interstitial nephritis: a brief review. *Am J Pathol.* 1976; 83:214–36.

372. Herbert V. Legal aspects of specious dietary claims. *Bull NY Acad Med.* 1982; 58:242–53.

373. Hernberg S, Laamanen A. Results of diagnostic lead mobilization tests in a Finnish series. *Ann Med Intern Fenn.* 1964; 53:123–28.

374. Hill J. *A History of Materia Medica.* London: T Longman, C Hitch, L Hawes, 1751.

375. Hillary W. *Observations on the Changes in the Air, and the Concomitant Epidemial Diseases in the Island of Barbados.* 2nd ed. London: L Hawes, W Clark, R Collins, 1766.

376. Hirschfeld E. Angina pectoris saturnina. *Klin Med.* 1926; 104:598–712.

377. Hoffa A. *Ueber Nephritis Saturnina.* Inaugural dissertation. Freiburg: Wagner, 1883.

378. Hoffman IF. *Fundamenta Medicinae* (1695). Translated by L King. New York: American Elsevier, 1971.

379. Holbrook SH. *The Golden Age of Quackery.* New York: Macmillan, 1959.

380. Hollander E. *Die Medizin in der Klassischer Malerie.* Stuttgart: Ferdinand Enke, 1923.

381. Home F. *Clinical Experiments, Histories, and Dissections.* 2nd ed. London: J Murray, 1782.

382. Hong CD, Hanenson IB, Lerner S, Hammond PB, Pesce AJ, Pollak VE. Occupational exposure to lead: effects on renal function. *Kidney Int.* 1980; 18:489–94.

383. Hong CD, Pollak VE, Pesce AJ, Hanenson IB, Brooks S. Proximal renal tubular dysfunction in asymptomatic occupational lead poisoning. *Kidney Int.* 1978; 14:654.

384. Hood P. *A Treatise on Gout, Rheumatism and Allied Afflictions.* Philadelphia: J and A Churchill, 1879.

385. Howship J. *A Practical Treatise on the Symptoms, Causes, Discrimination, and Treatment of Some of the Most Important Complaints that Affect the Secretion and Excretion of the Urine.* London: Longman, Hurst, Rees, Orme, Brown, 1823.

386. Hug R. Bleivergiftung und porphyrie. *Schweiz Med Wochenschr.* 1946; 76:322–24.

387. Hunt J. *Salutary Cautions Respecting the Gout in which the Doctrines Maintained in a Recent Publication by Dr Kinglake are Exposed and Refuted.* London: R Taylor, 1805.

388. Hunter J. Some experiments made upon rum, in order to ascertain the

cause of the colic, frequent among the soldiers in the Island of Jamaica, in the years 1781 and 1782. *Med Tr, Lond.* 1785; 3:227–49.

389. Hutchinson JH. Cirrhosis of the kidneys from lead poisoning. *Tr Pathol Soc, Phil.* 1877; 6:102–3.

390. Huxham J. *Observations on the Air and Epidemic Diseases from the Years 1728–1738, together with a Short Dissertation on the Devonshire Colic.* London: J Hinton, 1759.

391. Inglis JA, Henderson DA, Emmerson BT. The pathology and pathogenesis of chronic lead nephropathy occurring in Queensland. *J Pathol.* 1978; 124:65–76.

392. Ingram D. *An Essay on the Cause and Seat of the Gout.* Reading: J Newbery, C Micklewright, 1743.

393. Ireland GH. *The Preventable Causes of Disease, Injury and Death in American Manufactories and Workshops, and the Best Means and Appliances for Preventing and Avoiding Them.* Lomb Prize Essay at the American Public Health Association, Concord, NH: Republican Press Association, 1886.

394. Jaccoud S. Cardiopathie complexe et néphrite par l'intoxication plombique. *Rev Practique Travaux Med.* 1897:369–71.

395. Jacobson KH. Blood lead. *J Occup Med.* 1975; 17:413.

396. James R. *A Medical Dictionary.* London: T Osborne, 1743.

397. ———. *The Modern Practice of Physic . . .* Vol 2. London: J Hodges, 1746.

398. Janeway TC. Nephritic hypertension—clinical and experimental studies. *Harvey Lectures.* 1912–13:208–51.

399. Jarcho S. Some lost, obsolete, or discontinued diseases: serous apoplexy, incubus, and retrocedent ailments. *Tr Stud Cell Phys.* 1980; 2:241–66.

400. Jeans T. *A treatise on the Gout . . .* London: T Cadell, 1792.

401. Jendrassik E. Das Calomel als Diureticum. *Deutsch Arch Klin Med.* 1886; 38:499–524.

402. Jeremy R. Should asymptomatic hyperurecemia be treated? *Med J Aust.* 1972; 2:505–6.

403. Jhaveri R, Lavorgna L, Dube SK, Glass L, Khan F, Evans H. Relationship of blood pressure to lead concentration in small children. *Pediatrics.* 1979; 63:674–76.

404. Johannes XXI (Pope). *The Treasury of Healthe.* 1560.

405. Johnson G. *On the Diseases of the Kidney, their Pathology, Diagnosis and Treatment.* London: JW Parker and Son, 1852.

406. ———. *The Pathology of the Contracted Kidney and the Associated Cardio-Arterial Changes.* London: J and A Churchill, 1896.

407. Johnson J. *The Influence of the Atmosphere more Especially the Atmosphere of the British Isles on the Health Functions of the Human Frame.* London: T and C Underwood, Highley and Son, 1818.

408. Johnstone RT. Clinical inorganic lead intoxication. *Arch Environ Health.* 1964; 8:250–55.

409. Jones EC. *An Account of the Remarkable Effects of the Eau medicinale d'Husson in the Gout.* London: White and Cochrane, 1810.

410. Jores L. Ueber die pathologische Anatomie der chronischen Bleivergiftung des Kaninchens. *Beitr Pathol Anat.* 1902; 31:183–216.
411. Kaelbling R, Craig JR, Pasamnick B. Urinary porphobilinogen: results of screening 2,500 psychiatric patients. *Arch Gen Psych (Chi).* 1961; 5:494–508.
412. Karai I, Fukumoto K, Horiguchi S. An increase in Na⁺ K⁺–ATP-ase activity of erythrocyte membranes in workers employed in a lead refining factory. *Brit J Industr Med.* 1982; 39:290–94.
413. Katz WA. Deposition of urate crystals in gout: altered connective tissue metabolism. *Arthritis Rheum.* 1975; 18:751–56.
414. Kelleher K. The gout doctor: George Cheyne MD (1671–1743). *Practitioner.* 1971; 206:416–21.
415. Kelley WN, Weiner IM, eds. *Uric Acid. Handbook of Experimental Pharmacology.* Vol. 51. New York: Springer-Verlag, 1978.
416. Kellner E. *Moonshine: Its History and Folklore.* New York: Bobbs-Merill Co, 1971.
417. Kemp JA. Chronic lead poisoning. *J M A Georgia.* 1959; 2:468–73.
418. King LS. *The Medical World of the Eighteenth Century.* Chicago: Univ. of Chicago Press, 1958.
419. King-Hele D. *Erasmus Darwin.* New York: Charles Scribner's Sons, 1963.
420. Kinglake R. *Dissertation on Gout . . .* London: John Murray, 1804.
421. Kinnel J, Haden R. Gout: a review of 62 cases. *Med Clin North Am.* 1940; 24–28:429–41.
422. Klein M, Namer R, Harpur E, Corbin R. Earthenware containers as a source of fatal lead poisoning: case study and public health considerations. *N Engl J Med.* 1970; 283:669–72.
423. Klinenberg JR. Saturnine gout—a moonshine malady. *N Engl J Med.* 1969; 280:1238–39.
424. Klinenberg Jr, Bluestone R, Schlosstein L, Waisman J, Whitehouse NW. Urate deposition disease. *Ann Intern Med.* 1973; 78:99–111.
425. Klinenberg JR, Gonick HC, Dornfeld L. Renal function abnormalities in patients with asymptomatic hyperuricemia. *Acta Rheum.* 1975; 18:723–30.
426. Klinenberg JR, Kippen I, Bluestone R. Hyperuricemic nephropathy: pathologic features and factors influencing urate deposition. *Nephron.* 1975; 14:88–98.
427. Kolbel F, Gregorova I, Sonka J. Hyperuricaemia in hypertension. *Lancet.* 1965; i:519–20.
428. Koller K, Zollinger HU. Klinik und Laboratorium: Gichtische Glomerulosklerose. *Schweiz Med Wochenscher.* 1945; 75:97–105.
429. Koller LD, Brauner JA. Decreased B-lymphocyte response after exposure to lead and cadmium. *Toxicol Appl Pharmacol.* 1977; 44:621–24.
430. Koller LD, Kovacic S. Decreased antibody formation in mice exposed to lead. *Nature.* 1974; 250:148–49.
431. Kreimer-Birnbaum M, Grinstein M. Porphyrin biosynthesis. III. Porphyrin metabolism in experimental lead poisoning. *Biochim Biophys Acta.* 1965; 111:110–23.
432. Kuzell WC, Schaffarzick RW, Naugler WE, Koets P, Mankle EA, Brown B,

Champlin B. Some observations on 520 gouty patients. *J Chronic Dis.* 1955; 2:645–49.

433. "Lady A." *The Doctor Dissected or Willy Cadogen in the Kitchen.* London: T Davies and S Leacroft, 1771.

434. Laidlaw W. Remarks on the internal exhibition of the acetate of lead, chiefly with the view of determining to what extent it may be safely administered in the cure of diseases, especially in uterine haemorrhages. *Boston Med Surg J.* 1828–29; 1:147–52.

435. Lambe W. *Researches into the Properties of Spring Water with Medical Cautions (Illustrated by Cases) Against the Use of Lead in the Construction of Pumps, Water-Pipes, Cisterns &c.* London: J Johnson, 1803.

436. Lancereaux E. Note relative a un cas de paralysie saturnine avec altération des cordons nerveux et des muscles paralysés. *Gaz Med de Paris.* 1862; 17:709–13.

437. ———. De l'altération des reins dans l'intoxication saturnine. *L'Union Med.* 1863; 20:513–22.

438. ———. Saturnisme chronique avec accès de goutte et arthrites uratiques. *Compt Rend Soc de Biol, Par.* 1872; 2:99–106.

439. ———. Néphrite et arthrite saturnines: coincidence de ces affections: parallèle avec la néphrite et l'arthrite goutteuses. *Arch Gen de Med, Par.* 1881; 6:641–53.

440. ———. Nephritis and lead poisoning. *Med Press.* 1892; 5:422–24.

441. Landrigan PJ, Albrecht WN, Watanabe A, Lee S. *Health Hazard Evaluation Report: Ferro Corporation, Cleveland, Ohio.* National Institute of Occupational Safety and Health, Hazard Evaluation and Technical Assistance Branch. 1981. HETA 80-116.

442. Lane CR, Lawrence A. Home-made wine as a cause of lead poisoning: report of a case. *Br Med J.* 1961; 2:939–40.

443. Lane RE. The care of the lead worker. *Br J Ind Med.* 1949; 6:125–43.

444. ———. The clinical aspects of poisoning by inorganic lead components. *Ann Occup Hyg.* 1965; 8:31–34.

445. Latham J. *Facts and Opinions Concerning Diabetes.* London: John Murray, 1811.

446. Lavrand H. La néphrite des saturnins. *L'Oeuvre Med Chir.* 1899; 13:1–39.

447. Lawall CH. *Four Thousand Years of Pharmacy . . .* Philadelphia: JB Lippincott, 1927.

448. Leckie WJH, Tomsett SL. The diagnostic and therapeutic use of edathanil calcium disodium (EDTA Versene) in excessive inorganic lead absorption. *Q J Med.* 1958; 27:65–82.

449. Lecorché. *Traité des maladies des reins et des altérations pathologique de l'urine.* Paris: G Masson, 1875.

450. Lee W. *The Use of Brandy and Salt as a Remedy for Various Internal as well as External Diseases, Inflammation and Local Injuries.* Boston: CCP Moody, 1851.

451. Leeuwenhoek, van, A. An abstract of a letter from Mr. Leewenhoeck, to the R.S. dated Jan 23rd, 1684/5, concerning the various figures of the salts contained in several substances. *Philosoph Tr.* 1685; 173:1067–92.

452. Legge TM. *Industrial Maladies*. London: H Milford, Oxford Univ. Press, 1934.
453. Legge TM, Goadby KW. *Lead Poisoning and Lead Absorption*. New York: Longmans, Green and Co, 1912.
454. Lejeune E, Tolot F, Meunier, P. Goutte et hyperuricémie au cours du saturnisme. *Rev Rhum Mal Osteoartic.* 1969; 36:161–73.
455. Lemery N. *A Course of Chymistry*. 5th ed. Translated by W Harris. London: RN for Walter Kettilby, 1686.
456. Lenoble E, Daniel F. Constatation du plomb dans un rein saturnin un mois après la cessation de l'intoxication professionnelle. *Bull Mem Soc Med Hop de Paris.* 1918; 3:277–79.
457. Lerner S. Blood lead. *J Occup Med.* 1975; 17:413.
458. Levin NW, Abrahams OL. Allopurinol in patients with impaired renal function. *Ann Rheum Dis.* 1966; 25:681–87.
459. Lewis W. *The New Dispensatory*. London: J Nourse, 1753.
460. Leyden. Ein Fall von Bleivergiftung. *Z Klin Med.* 1883; 7:85–90.
461. Lichtenstein L, Scott HW, Levin MH. Pathologic changes in gout: survey of eleven necropsied cases. *Am J Pathol.* 1956; 32:871–95.
462. Lieb J, Hershman D. Isaac Newton: mercury poisoning or manic depression. *Lancet.* 1983; ii:1479–80.
463. Lieber CS, Jones DP, Losowsky MS, Davidson CS. Interrelation of uric acid and ethanol metabolism in man. *J Clin Invest.* 1962; 41:1863–70.
464. Lightfoote J, Blair HJ, Cohen JR. Lead intoxication in an adult caused by Chinese herbal medication. *JAMA.* 1977; 238:1539.
465. Lilis R, Dumitriu C, Roventa R, Nestorescu B, Pilat L. Renal function in chronic lead poisoning. *Med Lav.* 1967; 58:506–12.
466. Lilis R, Fischbein A, Valciukas JA, Blumberg W, Selikoff IJ. Kidney function and lead: relationships in several occupational groups with different levels of exposure. *Am J Indust Med.* 1980; 1:405–12.
467. ———. Renal function impairment in lead exposed worker: correlations with zinc protoporphyrins and blood lead levels. In: B Holmstead, R Lauwerys, M Mercier, M Robesfroid, eds. *Mechanisms of Toxicity and Hazard Evaluation*. New York: Elsevier/North Holland Biomedical Press, 1980.
468. Lilis R, Garilescu N, Nestoresca C, Dumitriu C, Roventa A. Nephropathy in chronic lead poisoning. *Br J Indust Med.* 1968; 25:196–202.
469. Lilis R, Valciukas J, Fischbein A, Andrews G, Selikoff IJ, Blumberg W. Renal function impairment in secondary lead smelter workers: correlations with zinc protoporphyrins and blood lead levels. *J Environ Pathol Toxicol.* 1979; 2:1447–74.
470. Lilis R, Valciukas JA, Sarcosi L, Campbell C, Selikoff IJ. Assessment of lead health hazards in a body shop at an automobile assembly plant. *Am J Indust Med.* 1982; 3:33–51.
471. Lindeboom GA. *Hermann Boerhaave: The Man and His Work*. London: Methuen and Co, 1968.
472. Linduff KM. The incidence of lead in late Shang and early Chou ritual vessels. *Expedition.* 1977; 19:7–16.

473. Linnane JW, Burry AF, Emmerson BT. Urate deposits in the renal medulla. *Nephron.* 1978; 29:216–22.

474. Long ER. *Selected Readings in Pathology.* 2nd ed. Springfield: Charles C Thomas, 1961.

475. Long M. Report of a committee of the centre district of the Medical Society of New Hampshire, on some recent cases of colica pictonum in Concord, N.H. *N Engl J Med Surg.* 1823; 12:255–58.

476. Lorimer G. Saturnine gout, and its distinguishing marks.*Br Med J.* 1886; 2:163.

477. Luckey WN. Remarks on some uncommonly violent cases of "Colica pictonum." *Am Med Rec.* 1818; 1:501–6.

478. Ludwig H. Saturnine gout: a secondary type of gout. *Arch Intern Med.* 1957; 100:802–12.

479. Luft FC, Weinburger MH, Grim CE. Sodium sensitivity and resistance in normotensive humans. *Am J Med.* 1982; 72:726–36.

480. Luthje H. Ueber Bleigicht und den Einfluss der Bleiintoxication auf der Harnsaureausscheidung. *Klin Med.* 1896; 29:266–323.

481. Macalpine I, Hunter R. The "insanity" of George III: a classic case of porphyria. *Brit Med J.* 1966; 1:65–71.

482. Macalpine I, Hunter R, Rimington C. Porphyria in the royal houses of Stuart, Hanover and Prussia: a follow-up study of George III's illness. *Brit Med J.* 1968; 1:7–18.

483. McAllister RG, Michelakis AM, Sandstead HH. Plasma renin activity in chronic plumbism. *Arch Int Med.* 1971; 127:919–23.

484. McCarthy DJ. A historical note: Leeuwenhoek's description of crystals from a gouty tophus. *Arthritis Rheum.* 1970; 13:414–18.

485. ———. The gouty toe—a multifactorial condition. *Ann Intern Med.* 1977; 86:234–36.

486. McConaghey RMS. Sir George Baker and the Devonshire colic. *Med Hist.* 1967; 11:345–60.

487. McCord CP. Lead and lead poisoning in early America: Benjamin Franklin and lead poisoning. *Ind Med Surg J.* 1953; 22:393–99.

488. ———. Lead and lead poisoning in early America: the pewter era. *Ind Med Sug J.* 1953; 22:573–77.

489. McCready BW. *On the Influence of Trades, Professions, and Occupations in the United States, in the Production of Disease.* Baltimore: Johns Hopkins Univ. Press, 1943.

490. Macdonnell. Chronic lead poisoning. *Montreal Hosp Rep.* 1889; 18:291–94.

491. McKhann CF. Lead poisoning in children. *Am J Dis Child.* 1926; 32:386–92.

492. Maclachlan MJ, Rodnan GP. Effects of food, fast and alcohol on serum uric acid and acute attacks of gout. *Am J Med.* 1967; 42:38.

493. McMichael AJ, Johnson HM. Long-term mortality profile of heavily-exposed lead smelter workers. *J Occup Med.* 1982; 24:375–78.

494. Macmichael W. *The Gold-Headed Cane.* 2nd ed. 1827. Reprint. New York: Paul B Hoeber, 1915.

495. McNeil JR, Reinhard MC. Lead poisoning from home remedies. *Clin Ped.* 1967; 6:150–56.

496. McQueen EG. The syndrome of gout. *Med J Aust.* 1951; 5:644–50.

497. Magendie F. *Summary of Physiology.* Translated by J Revere. Baltimore: EJ Cooke, 1822.

498. Maggioni G, Bottini E, Biagi G. Contributo alla conoscenza dell'amino-aciduria qualitativa e quantitativa nell'intossicazione da piombo nel bambino. *Boll Soc Ital Biol Sper.* 1960; 36:193–96.

499. Magid E, Hilden M. Elevated levels of blood lead in alcoholic liver disease. *Int Arch Occup Health.* 1975; 35:61–65.

500. Mahaffey KR, Annest JL, Roberts J, Murphy RS. National estimates of blood lead levels: United States, 1976–1980. Association with selected demographic and socioeconomic factors. *N Engl J Med.* 1982; 307:573–79.

501. Mahomed FA. On chronic Bright's disease, and its essential symptoms. *Lancet.* 1879; i:46–47, 76–78, 149–50, 261–63, 399–401, 437–38.

502. ———. Some of the clinical aspects of chronic Bright's disease. *Guy's Hosp Rep., Par.* 1879; 24:363–436.

503. ———. Chronic Bright's disease without albuminuria. *Guy's Hosp Rep, Par.* 1881; 3:295–416.

504. Mahot B. Saturnisme; goutte saturnine: néphrite interstitielle—accidents urémiques—mort—autopsie. *Gaz Hop.* 1877:186–88.

505. Maimonides M. *Treatise on Poisons and Their Antidotes.* Muntner S, ed. Philadelphia: JB Lippincott Co, 1966.

506. Major RH. *A History of Medicine.* Springfield: Charles C Thomas, 1954.

507. Malcolm D. Precautions for lead workers. *Practitioner.* 1971; 207:211.

508. ———. Prevention of long term sequelae following the absorption of lead. *Arch Environ Health.* 1971; 23:292–98.

509. Malcolm D, Barnett HAR. A mortality study of lead workers 1925–1976. *Brit J Indust Med.* 1982; 39:404–10.

510. Mann J. *Medical Sketches of the Campaigns of 1812, 13, 14 . . .* Dedham: H Mann and Co, 1816.

511. ———. Practical observations on colica Pictonum. *N Engl J Med Surg.* 1822; 11:17–21.

512. Marsh WA. Saturnine gout. *Guy's Hosp Rep, Par.* 1870; 15:42–46.

513. Marshall E. EPA faults classic lead study. *Science.* 1983; 222:906–7.

514. Marshall W. *The Rural Economy of the West of England Including Devonshire . . .* Dublin: P Wogan, P Byrne, J Rice and J Moore, 1797.

515. Marten J. *The Dishonour of the Gout: or a serious answer to a Ludicrous Pamphlet . . .* London: J Isted, 1737.

516. Mather C. *The Angel of Bethesda.* Jones GW, ed. Barre: Am Antiquarian Soc and Barre Publishing Co, 1972.

517. Mathieu A, Malibran. Saturnisme; hémorragies cérébrale et bulbaire; hémiplégie et paralysie des extenseurs du même côté. Hypertrophie du ventricule gauche, néphrite interstitielle, albuminurie. *Le Progres Med.* 1884; 12:827–28.

518. Matthissen HG. *De lithargyrio infectis et colica par etico convulsiva ex-*

haustu corundum oriunda. Unpublished translation by M Sollenberger. Griefswald: Hieronymas Johannes Struck, 1745.

519. Mayerne, De, T. *A Treatise on the Gout*. Translated by T Sherley. London: D Newman, 1676.

520. Mayers M. A study of the lead line, arteriosclerosis and hypertension in 381 lead workers. *J Ind Hyg*. 1927; 9:239.

521. Mayers MR. Industrial lead exposure. *J Occup Med*. 1947; 3:77–83.

522. Mayne JG. Pathological study of the renal lesions found in 27 patients with gout. *Ann Rheum Dis*. 1955; 15:61.

523. Mead R. *A Mechanical Account of Poisons, in Several Essays*. 3rd ed. London: J Brindley, 1745.

524. Meiklejohn A. The Millreek and the Devonshire colic. *Br J Indust Med*. 1954; 11:40–44.

525. ———. The successful prevention of lead poisoning in the glazing of earthenware in the North Staffordshire potteries. *Brit J Indust Med*. 1963; 20:169–80.

526. Menetrier P. Encéphalopathie saturnine et hypertension artérielle. *Bull Mem Soc Med Hop de Paris*. 1904; 31:141–47.

527. Messerli FH, Frohlich ED, Dreslinski GR, Suarez DH, Aristimuno GG. Serum uric acid in essential hypertension: an indicator of renal vascular involvement. *Ann Intern Med*. 1980; 93:817–21.

528. Minden H. Die Beteiligung des Gefasssystems bei Bleivergiftung. *Int Arch Gewerbepath u Gewerbehyg*. 1962; 19:581–88.

529. Mirouze J, Miton C, Mathieu-Daude P, Monnier L, Selam JL. Néphropathie chronique au cours d'un saturmisme. *Nouv Presse Med*. 1975; 4:1642–44.

530. Misaurius P (pseudonym). *The Honour of the Gout*. London: R Gosling, 1735.

531. Modern FWS, Meister L. The kidney of gout, a clinical entity. *Med Clin North Am*. 1942; 36:941–51.

532. Moore J. *A letter to Dr Jones on the composition of the Eau Medicinale d'Husson*. London: J Johnson, 1811.

533. Moore N. Some observations on the morbid anatomy of gout. *St Bartholomew's Hosp Rep*. 1887; 23:289–344.

534. Morgan JM. A simplified screening test for exposure to lead. *South Med J*. 1967; 60:435.

535. ———. The consequences of chronic lead exposure. *Ala J Med Sci*. 1968; 5:454–57.

536. ———. Chelation therapy in lead nephropathy. *South Med J*. 1975; 68:1001–6.

537. ———. Hyperkalemia and acidosis in lead nephropathy. *South Med J*. 1976; 69:881–86.

538. Morgan JM, Burch HB. Comparative tests for diagnosis of lead poisoning. *Arch Intern Med*. 1972; 130:335–40.

539. Morgan JM, Hartley MW. Etiologic factors in lead nephropathy. *South Med J*. 1976; 69:1445–49.

540. Morgen J. "Normal" lead and cadmium content of the human kidney. *Arch Environ Health*. 1972; 24:364–68.

541. Mosely B. *A Treatise on Tropical Diseases on Military Operations and on the Climate of the West Indies.* London: Nichols and Son, 1803.

542. Mouw DR, Wagner JG, Kalitis K, Vander AJ, Mayor GH. The effect of parathyroid hormone on the renal accumulation of lead. *Environ Res.* 1978; 15:20–27.

543. Murray RE. *Plumbism and Chronic Nephritis in Young People in Queensland. Commonwealth of Australia: Department of Health Publication Number 2.* Sydney: Univ. of Sydney, 1939.

544. *National Geographic.* That noble river, the Thames. 1983; 163:760–87.

545. National Research Council. *Airborne Lead in Perspective.* Committee on Biological effects of Atmospheric Polutants. Washington, DC: National Academy of Sciences, 1972.

546. ———. *Lead in the Human Environment.* A report prepared by the Committee on Lead in the Human Environment. Washington, DC: National Academy of Sciences, 1980.

547. Needleman HL. *Low Level Lead Exposure.* New York: Raven Press, 1980.

548. Neilan BA, Taddeini CE, McJilton, Handwerger BS. Decreased T cell function in mice exposed to chronic, low levels of lead. *Clin Exp Immunol.* 1980; 39:746–49.

549. Nelken D. Workers at risk. *Science.* 1983; 222:125.

550. Neumann C. *Chemical Works.* London: W Johnston, 1759.

551. Newcombe DS. Gouty arthritis and polycystic kidney disease. *Ann Intern Med.* 1973; 79:605.

552. Nicander. *Alexpharmica.* Unpublished translation by M Sollenberger. O. Schmeider, ed. Leipzig, 1856.

553. Nordberg GF, ed. *Effects and Dose-Response Relationships of the Toxic Metals.* New York: Elsevier Scientific Publishing Co, 1976.

554. Nriagu JO. *Lead and Lead Poisoning in Antiquity.* New York: John Wiley, 1983.

555. ———. Saturnine gout among Roman aristocrats. *N Engl J Med.* 1983; 308:660–63.

556. Nye LJJ. An investigation of the extraordinary incidence of chronic nephritis in young people in Queensland. *Med J Aust.* 1929; 2:145–59.

557. ———. *Chronic Nephritis and Lead Poisoning.* Sydney: Angus and Robertson, 1933.

558. Ogryzlo MA. Hyperuricemia induced by high fat diets and starvation. *Arthritis Rheum.* 1965; 8:799–818.

559. ———. Effects of allopurinol on gouty and non-gouty uric acid nephropathy. *Ann Rheum Dis.* 1966; 25:673–80.

560. Oleson CW. *Secret Nostrums and Systems of Medicine. A Book of Formulas.* 7th ed. Chicago: Oleson and Co, 1899.

561. Oliver G. *A Contribution to the Study of the Blood and Blood-Pressure.* London: HK Lewis, 1901.

562. ———. *Lead Poisoning in its Acute and Chronic Forms.* London: Young J Pentland, 1891.

563. ———. *Diseases of Occupation from the Legislative, Social and Medical Points of View.* New York: EP Dutton and Co, 1908.

564. ———. *Lead Poisoning from the Industrial, Medical and Social Points of View.* New York: Paul B Hoeber, 1914.

565. Oliver W. *A Practical Dissertation on Bath Waters.* 4th ed. London: James Leake, 1747.

566. Ollivier A. Report médico-légal sur les accidens aprovés par les plaignans. *Ann d'hyg, Par.* 1842; 27:113–18.

567. ———. De l'albuminurie saturnine. *Arch gen de med, Par.* 1863; 2:530–46.

568. ———. Nombreuses coliques de plomb: accès épileptiformes: albuminurie persistante et très-prononcé: atrophie musculaire progressive. Mort avec des symptomes d'asphyxie. Autopsie:néphrite parenchymateuse. *Compt Rend Soc de Biol, Par.* 1865; 4:127–30.

569. Olsen F. Transfer of arterial hypertension by splenic cells from doca-salt hypertensive and renal hypertensive rats to normotensive recipients. *Acta Path Microbiol Scand.* 1980; 88:1–5.

570. Ophuls W. Experimental chronic nephritis. *JAMA.* 1907; 48:483–90.

571. ———. Chronic lead poisoning in guinea pigs: with special reference to nephritis, cirrhosis and polyneuritis. *Ann J Med Sci.* 1915; 150:518–41.

572. Orfila MP. *Popular Treatise on the Remedies to be Employed in Cases of Poisoning and Apparent Death: Including the Means of Detecting Poisons, of Distinguishing Real from Apparent Death and of Ascertaining the Adulteration of Wines.* Translated by W Price. Philadelphia: Solomon W Conrad, 1818.

573. Osborne J. *On the Nature and Treatment of Dropsical Diseases.* London: Sherwood, Gilbert and Piper, 1837.

574. Osler W. *The Principles and Practice of Medicine.* 7th ed. New York: D Appleton and Co, 1910.

575. Ostberg Y. Renal urate deposits in chronic renal insufficiency. *Acta Med Scand.* 1968; 183:197–201.

576. Packard FA. A small series of cases of lead poisoning, with remarks upon saturnine gout. *Phil Hosp Rep.* 1896; 3:29–44.

577. Packard FP. *History of Medicine in the United States.* New York: Paul B Hoeber, 1931.

578. Padilla F. Effect of chronic lead intoxication on blood pressure in the rat. *Am J Med Sci.* 1969; 258:359.

579. Page GR. Some of the effects of chronic lead poisoning, with special reference to arteriosclerosis. *J State Med, Lond.* 1921; 39:161–68.

580. Pagel W. *Paracelsus. An Introduction to Philosophical Medicine in the Era of the Renaissance.* New York: S Karger, 1958.

581. Paillard H. La goutte par insuffisance rénale. *J Med Franc.* 1949; 162:23–26.

582. Pansa M. *Consilium Antipodagracum Specialisimum. Der dritte Theil der Gicht Bucher. . . . Appendix X. Consilia Specia Lissima.* Leipzig: Thomas Scharers, 1623.

583. Paracelsus. *The Hermetic and Alchemical Writings of Aureolus Philippus Theophrastus Bombast, of Hohenheim, Called Paracelsus the Great.* Vol II. Waite AE, ed. Berkeley: Shambhala, 1976.

584. Pardo V, Perez-Stable E, Fisher ER. Ultrastructural studies in hypertension. III. Gouty nephropathy. *Lab Invest.* 1968; 18:143–50.

585. Parelle E. *De la Pseudo-Paralysie Générale Saturnine.* Paris: G Stoneheil, 1889.

586. Parkin J. *On Gout: Its Cause, Nature and Treatment.* London: John Hatchard and Son, 1841.

587. Parkinson J. *Observations on the Nature and Cure of Gout . . .* London: C Whittingham, 1805.

588. Parry CH. *Collection From the Unpublished Writings of the Late Caleb Hillier Parry, MD.* London: Underwoods, 1825.

589. Pasteur-Vallery-Radot, Derot M. Les néphrites saturnines. *Paris Med.* 1930:341–45.

590. Patterson CC. Native copper, silver, and gold accessible to early metallurgists. *American Antiquity.* 1971; 36:286–321.

591. Patterson M, Jernigan WCI. Lead intoxication from "moonshine". *GP.* 1969; 40:126–30.

592. Pechey J. *A Collection of Chronical Disease: viz the Colick; the Bilious Colick; Hysterick Diseases. The Gout; and the Bloody Urine from the Stone in the Kidnies.* London: Henry Bostwicke, 1693.

593. Pecora L. Porphyrie cutanée et saturnisme. *La Presse Med.* 1969; 77:1192.

594. Pedell. Wahre Gicht mit Nierenschrunptung bei Bleiintoxication. *Dtsch Med Wochenschr.* 1884; 9:9.

595. Pejic S. The nature of the primary renal lesion produced by lead. *Ann Intern Med.* 1928; 1:577–604.

596. Pemberton CR. *A Practical Treatise on Various Diseases of the Abdominal Viscera.* 1st ed. 1806. Worcester: GA Trumbull, 1815.

597. Percival T. *Observations and Experiments on the Poison of Lead.* London: J Johnson, 1774.

598. ———. *Essays Medical, Philophical and Experimental.* 4th ed. Warrington: W. Eyres, 1788.

599. Perry W. *A Dialogue in the Shades, Recommended to Every Purchaser of Dr. Kinglake's Dissertation . . .* Uxbridge: T Lake, 1805.

600. Peters HA. Chelation therapy in acute, chronic and mixed porphyria. In: MJ Seven, LA Johnson, eds. *Metal-Binding in Medicine.* Philadelphia: JB Lippincott Co, 1960.

601. Pettigrew TJ. *On Superstitions Connected with the History and Practice of Medicine and Surgery.* Philadelphia: E Barrington and GD Haswell, 1844.

602. Philips J. Cyder. In: *The Works of the English Poets with Prefaces Biographical and Critical by Samuel Johnson.* London: H Hughs, 1779.

603. Pierce R. *Bath Memoires.* Bristol: D Hammond, 1697.

604. Ping-Yu H, Needham J. Elixir poisoning in medieval China. *Janus.* 1959:221–45.

605. Piomelli S, Seaman C, Zullow D, Curran A, Davidow B. Threshold for lead damage to heme synthesis in urban children. *Proc Natl Acad Sci.* 1982; 79:3335–39.

606. Piper WN, Tephly TR. Differential inhibition of erythrocyte and hepatic uroporphyrinogen I synthetase activity by lead. *Life Sci.* 1974; 14:873–76.

607. Plinius C. *The Historie of the World commonly called the Natural Historie of C Plinius Secundus.* Vol II. Translated by P Holland. London: Adam Islip, 1634.

608. Popert, Hewitt JV. Gout and hyperuricemia in rural and urban populations. *Ann Rheum Dis.* 1962; 21:154–63.

609. Prerovska I, Teisinger J. Excretion of lead and its biological activity several years after termination of exposure. *Brit J Ind Med.* 1970; 27:352–55.

610. Prout W. *An Inquiry into the Nature and Treatment of Diabetes, Calculous and other Affections of the Urinary Organs . . .* Philadelphia: Towar and Hogan, 1826.

611. Pueschel SM, Kapito L, Schwachman H. Children with an increased lead burden: a screening and follow up study. *JAMA.* 1972; 222:462–66.

612. Purcell J. *A Treatise of the Cholick . . .* London: W Lewis, 1714.

613. Putman JJ. On the frequency with which lead is found in the urine, and on certain points in the symptomatology of chronic lead poisoning. *Boston Med Surg J.* 1887; 117:73–76.

614. Quier J. *Letters and Essays on the Small Pox and Innoculation, the Measels, the Dry-Belly-Ache . . . of the West Indies.* London: J. Murray, 1778.

615. Quincy J. *Medicina Statica: Being the Aphorisms of Sanctorius.* 4th ed. London: J Osborn and T Longman, 1728.

616. Radonić M, Županić V, Radošević Z. The renal changes in lead poisoning—a clinical bioptical correlation. *Excerpt Med.* 1963; 67:145.

617. Radošević Z, Šarić M, Beritić T, Knežerić J. The kidney in lead poisoning. *Br J Ind Med.* 1961; 18:222–30.

618. Radulescu IC, Dinischiotu GT, Maugsch C, Ionescu C, Teodorescu-Exarcu I. Recherches sur l'atteinte du rein dans le saturnisme industriel par l'étude du clearance de la créatinine et de l'urée. *Arch Mal Prof.* 1957; 18:125–37.

619. Rakow AB, Lieben J. Twenty-four cases of lead poisoning, ten years later. *Arch Environ Health.* 1968; 16:785–87.

620. Ramazzini B. *Diseases of Workers* (1700). Translated by WC Wright. New York: Hafner Pub Co, 1964.

621. Ramirez-Cervantes B, Embree JW, Hine CH, Nelson KW, Varner MO, Putnam RD. Health assessment of employees with different body burdens of lead. *J Occup Med.* 1978; 20:610–17.

622. Ramsay LE. Hyperuricaemia in hypertension: role of alcohol. *Br Med J.* 1979; 1:653–54.

623. Rapado A. Relationship between gout and arterial hypertension. In: Sperling O, De Vries A, Wyngaarden JB, eds. *Purine Metabolism in Man: Biochemistry and Pharmacology of Uric Acid Metabolism.* New York: Plenum Press, 1974.

624. Rathery F, Michel R. Néphrite suraigue. Anurie et mort consécutive à l'ingestion répétée de petites doses de sous-acétate de plomb. *Bull Mem Soc Med Hôp de Paris.* 1923; 47:962–73.

625. Rayer PFO. *Traité des Maladies des Reins.* Paris: JB Baillière, 1839–41.

626. Read JL, Williams JP. Lead myocarditis: report of a case. *Am Heart J*. 1952; 44:797–802.

627. Rees GO. *On the Analysis of the Blood and Urine in Health and Disease: and on the Treatment of Urinary Diseases*. 2nd ed. London: Longman, Brown, Green and Longmans, 1845.

628. Reiders F. Effects of intravenous disodium calcium ethylene-diamine tetra-acetate (Na$_2$CaEDTA) on urinary excretion of Pb, Fe, Cu and Zn, in man. *Fed Proc*. 1955; 14:382.

629. Reiders F, Dunnington WC, Brieger H. The efficacy of edathamil calcium disodium in the treatment of occupational lead poisoning. *Ind Med Surg J*. 1955; 24:195–202.

630. Reif MC, Constantiner A, Levitt MF. Chronic gouty nephropathy: a vanishing syndrome? *New Engl J Med*. 1981; 304:535–36.

631. Reisman D. *The Story of Medicine in the Middle Ages*. New York: Paul B Hoeber, 1932.

632. Rennie A. *Observations on Gout . . .* London: Underwood, 1825.

633. Reynolds PP, Knapp MJ, Baraf HSB, Holmes EW. Moonshine and lead. *Arthritis and Rheumatism*. 1983; 26:1057–64.

634. Richet G. Saturnisme et insuffissance rénale chronique. *Acta Klin Belg*. 1964; 19:1–4.

635. Richet G, Albahary G, Ardaillou R, Sultan C, Morel-Maroger A. Le rein du saturnisme chronique. *Rev Franc Etudes Clin Biol*. 1964; 9:188–96.

636. Richet G, Albahary C, Morel-Maroger L, Guillaume G, Galle, P. Les altérations rénales dans 23 cas de saturnisme professional. *Bull Soc Med Hop Paris*. 1966; 117:441–46.

637. Richet G, Ardaillou R, Montera H, Slama R, Bougault T. Le rein goutteux. *Nouv Presse Med*. 1961; 69:644.

638. Richet G, Mignon F, Ardaillou R. Goutte secondaire des néphropathies chroniques. *Nouv Presse Med*. 1965; 73:633–38.

639. Riddell WR. Corradinus Gilinus and his Treatise de Morbo Gallico, 1497. *Med J Rec*. 1931; 134:434–55.

640. Rieke FE. Lead intoxication in shipbuilding and shipscraping—1941 to 1968. *Arch Environ Health*. 1969; 19:521–39.

641. Ring J. *A Treatise on the Gout*. London: B McMillan, 1811.

642. Riollay F. *A Letter to Dr Hardy, Physician, on the Hints He has Given Concerning the Origin of the Gout, in His Late Publication on the Devonshire Cholic*. Oxford: J and J Fletcher, 1778.

643. Riverius L. *The Practice of the Physic. In 17 Books*. Translated by N Culpeper. London: Peter Cole, 1655.

644. ———. *The Universal Body of Physick . . .* Translated by W Carr. London: Henry Eversden, 1657.

645. Rizzo A, Sbertoli C. La diagnosi della nefropatia saturnina alla luce della moderna fisiopatologia renale. *Med Lav*. 1956; 47:117–28.

646. Roberts W. *A Practical Treatise on Urinary and Renal Diseases, including Urinary Deposits*. Philadelphia: Henry C Lea, 1866.

647. Robertson WH. *The Nature and Treatment of Gout*. London: John Churchill, 1845.

648. Robinson N. *An Essay on the Gout . . .* London: Edward Robinson, 1755.
649. Rodnan GP. Early theories concerning the etiology and pathogenesis of the gout. *Arthritis Rheum.* 1965; 8:599–610.
650. Rodnan GP, Benedek TG. Ancient therapeutic arts in the gout. *Arthritis Rheum.* 1963; 6:317–40.
651. ———. Cotton Mather on rheumatism and the gout. *J Hist Med.* 1965; 20: 115–39.
652. Rollo J. *Cases of the Diabetes Mellitus . . .* 2nd ed. London: J Callow, 1806.
653. Roose R. *Gout and its Relations to Diseases of the Liver and Kidneys.* 6th ed. London: HK Lewis, 1889.
654. Rosen G. *The History of Miners' Disease.* New York: Schuman's, 1943.
655. Rosen JF, Chesney RW, Hamstra A, De Luca HF, Mahaffey KR. Reduction in 1,25-dihydroxy-vitamin D in children with increased lead absorption. *N Engl J Med.* 1980; 302:1128–31.
656. Rosenfeld JB. Effect of long-term allopurinol administration in normotensive and hypertensive hyperuricemic subjects. *Adv Exp Med Biol.* 1974; 41B:581–96.
657. Rossi L. La funzionalità renale nel saturnismo professionale. *La Riforma Med.* 1956; 70:841–51.
658. Roueche B. A perverse, ungrateful, maleficent malady. *New Yorker.* Mar. 13, 1948:67.
659. Rowley W. *A Treatise on the Regular, Irregular, Atonic and Flying Gout . . .* London: J Windgrave, E Newbery, T Hookham, 1792.
680. Rush B. An account of the efficacy of sugar of lead in curing epilepsy. *Phil Med Mus.* 1805; 1:60–61.
661. ———. *Medical Inquiries and Observations.* 2nd ed. Philadelphia: J Conrad and Co, 1805.
662. ———. *The Selected Writings of Benjamin Rush.* Vol 2. New York: Philosophical Library, 1947.
663. Saenger P, Rosen JF, Markowitz M. Diagnostic significance of edatate disodium testing in children with increased lead absorption. *Am J Dis Child.* 1982; 136:312–15.
664. Saker BM, Tofler DB, Burvill MJ, Reilly RA. Alcohol consumption and gout. *Med J Aust.* 1967; 1:1213–16.
665. Sale EP. Albuminuria—saturnine poisoning. *New Orleans J Med.* 1869:726–28.
666. Salmon W. *Synopsis Medicinae-Therapeutica . . .* Book 3. London: Thomas Dawks, 1680.
667. Sandstead HH, Mickelakis AM, Temple TE. Lead intoxication: its effect on the renin-aldosterone response to sodium deprivation. *Arch Environ Health.* 1970; 20:356–63.
668. Saundby R. The doctrine of saturnine gout. *Med Times Gaz.* 1881; 1:385–86.
669. Saunders W. *An Answer to the Observations of Mr. Geach, and to the Cursory Remarks of Dr. Alcock . . .* London: E and C Dillt, 1767.
670. Saylor RP, Wright LF. Is chronic plumbism important in pathogenesis of

renal disease in gout? *Abstracts: Am Soc Nephrol.* 15th Ann Meet, Chicago, IL, 1982:41 A.

671. Sayre LA. Three cases of lead palsy from the use of a cosmetic called "Laird's Bloom of Youth." *Tr AMA.* 1869.

672. Scheele KW. The chemical examination of urinary calculi. *Opuscula.* 1776; 2:73.

673. Schnitker MA. A history of the treatment of gout. *Bull Ind Hist Med.* 1936; 4:89.

674. Schnitker MA, Richter AB. Nephritis in gout. *Am J Med Sci.* 1936; 192:241–52.

675. Schroeder HA, Tipton IH. The human body burden of lead. *Arch Environ Health.* 1968; 17:965–78.

676. Scudamore C. *A Treatise on the Nature and Cure of Gout and Rheumatism . . .* 1st Am ed. Philadelphia: William Brown, 1819.

677. ———. *A Treatise on the Nature and Cure of Gout and Rheumatism . . .* 4th Engl ed. London: Joseph Mallett, 1823.

678. Semmes T. *An Essay on the Effects of Lead Comprising a Few Experiments on the Saccharum Saturnii and Its Application in the Cure of Diseases.* Philadelphia: Carr and Smith, 1801.

679. Sennert D, Culpeper N, Cole A. *Two Treatises. The First of the Venerial Pocks. . . . The Second of the Gout . . .* London: Peter Cole, 1660.

680. Sessa T, Guarino A. Su di un caso di miocardiopata saturnina: considerazioni diagnostiche e medico-legali. *Folia Med.* 1957; 40:273–99.

681. Settle DM, Patterson CC. Lead in albacore: guide to lead pollution in Americans. *Science.* 1980; 207:1167–76.

682. Shearman EJ. Two cases of lead poisoning with very large quantities of albumen in the urine. *Practitioner.* 1874–75; 12:266–68.

683. Short T. *The Natural, Experimental and Medicinal History of the Mineral Waters of Derbyshire, Lincolnshire and Yorkshire . . .* London: F Gyles, 1734.

684. ———. *Discourses on Tea, Sugar, Milk, Made Wines, Spirit, Punch, Tobacco, etc., with Plain and Useful Rules for Gouty People.* London: T Longman, A Millar, 1750.

685. Siemens, HJ. *Dissertatio Inauguralis Sistens Metallurgiam Morbiferam.* Unpublished translation by M. Sollenberger. Halle: Christian Henckel, 1695.

686. Siller WG. Avian nephritis and visceral gout. *Lab Invest.* 1969; 8:1319–49.

687. Simkin PA. The pathogenesis of podagra. *Ann Intern Med.* 1977; 86: 230–233.

688. Simmonds HA. Crystal induced nephropathy: a current view. *Eur J Rheum Inflamm.* 1978:86–91.

689. Smith D. *A Letter to Dr Cadogen with Remarks on the Most Interesting Paragraphs in His Treatise on the Gout . . .* 2nd ed. London: Carnas and Newbury, 1772.

690. Smith SA. Some aspect of lead absorption. *Med J Aust.* 1925; 11:391–94.

691. Smith WA. *Gout and the Gouty.* San Antonio: Naylor, 1970.

692. Sokoloff L. The pathology of gout. *Metabolism.* 1957; 6:230–43.

693. Solis-Cohen S. Cardiac disease (pancarditis) due to lead poisoning. *Int Clin.* 1901; 3:121–28.
694. Sorenson EMB, Moretti ES, Lindenbaum A. Chelation therapy and the tissue distribution and excretion of lead in mice. *Arch Environ Contam Toxicol.* 1980; 9:619–26.
695. Sorensen LB. The pathogenesis of gout. *Arch Intern Med.* 1962; 109: 55–66.
696. Spargo PE, Poands CA. Newton's derangement of the intellect: new light on an old problem. *Tr Royal Soc, Lond.* 1979; 34:11.
697. Specht W, Fischer K. Vergiftungsnachweis an den Resten einer Jahre alten Leiche. *Arch Kriminol.* 1959; 124:61–84.
698. Spence TRP. Account of sugar of lead, in a case of epilepsy. *Phil Med Museum.* 1806; 2:150–54.
699. Spencer HW, Yarger WE, Robinson RE. Alteration of renal function during dietary-induced hyperuricemia in the rat. *Kidney Int.* 1976; 9:489–500.
700. Spencer RH. Two cases of lead colic. *North West Med Surg J.* 1850; 6:467–69.
701. Spilberg I, Mandell B, Mehta J, Simchowitz L. Mechanism of action of colchicine in acute urate crystal-induced arthritis. *J Clin Invest.* 1979; 64: 75–780.
702. Spilsbury F. *Physical Dissertations on the Scurvy, and Gout . . .* London: J Wilkie, C Etherington, C Elliot, 1779.
703. ————. *Free Observations on the Scurvy, Gout, Diet and Remedy.* 3rd ed. London: Fisher, 1785.
704. Spring JA, Buss DH. Three centuries of alcohol in the British diet. *Nature, Lond.* 1977; 270:567–72.
705. Stearns S. *The American Herbal, or Materia Medica.* Walpole: David Carlisle, 1801.
706. Steele R. *Secreta Secretorum.* London: Kegan Paul, Trench, Trubner and Co, 1898.
707. Steele TH. Asymptomatic hyperuricemia: pathogenic or innocent bystander? *Arch Intern Med.* 1979; 139:24–25.
708. Steele TH, Reiselbach RE. The renal handling of urate and other organic anions. In: Brenner BM, Rector FC, eds. *The Kidney.* Philadelphia: WB Saunders Co, 1976:442–76.
709. Steinberg R. If you are highly sexed, achievement oriented, and a wine connoisseur, this may be your disease. The agonies and ecstasies of gout. *Esquire.* Feb. 13, 1979:80–81.
710. Stetten, DW, Jr. Aspects of the history and the natural history of gout. *Bull NJ Acad Med.* 1965; 11:7–18.
711. Stewart DD. Lead convulsions: a study of sixteen cases. *Am J Med Sci.* 1895; 109:288.
712. Stewart TG. *A Practical Treatise on Brights Diseases of the Kidneys.* New York: William Wood and Co, 1871.
713. Stockhausen PW. *Disertatio Inaugualis Medica Aegrum Exhibens Colica, Saturnina Laborantem.* Unpublished translation by M Sollenberger. Jena: Krebs, 1712.

714. Stockhausen S. *Traité des mauvais effets de la fumee de a litharge.* 1st ed. 1656. Paris: Ruault, 1776.

715. Stofen D. Environmental lead and the heart. *J Mol Cell Cardiol.* 1974; 6:285–90.

716. Stokvis BJ. Zur pathologenese der Hamatoporphyrinurie. *Klin Med.* 1895; 28:1–9.

717. Stone WJ. *Bright's Disease and Arterial Hypertension.* Philadelphia: WB Saunders, 1936.

718. Störck, von, A. *A Narrative of the Surprising Effects of the Meadow Saffron in the Cure of the Dropsy.* London: J Payne, 1766.

719. Strother E. *An Essay on Sickness and Health . . .* 2nd ed. London: Charles Rivington, 1725.

720. Stukeley WM. *Of the Gout . . .* London: J Roberts, 1734.

721. Sutton T. *Tracts on Delerium Tremens, or Peritonitis and on Some other Internal Inflammatory Affections and on the Gout.* London: Thomas Underwood, 1813.

722. Swieten, van, G. *An Abridgement of Baron Van Swieten's Commentaries Upon the Aphorisms of the Celebrated Dr Herman Boerhaave . . .* Translated by C Hossack. London: Robert Horsfield, 1773–75:28–55.

723. Sydenham T. *The Works of Thomas Sydenham . . .* Vol. 2. Translated by G Wallis. London: CGI and J Robinson, 1788.

724. ———. *The Works of Thomas Sydenham, 1683.* Translated by RG Latham. London: Sydenham Society, 1850.

725. Talbott JH. *Gout.* New York: Grune and Stratton, 1957.

726. ———. Clinical Experiences. *Arthritis Rheum.* 1975; 18:663–72.

727. Talbott JH, Lockie LM. Gouty arthritis. *Ciba Symposium.* 1950; 2: 319–57.

728. Talbott JH, Terplan KL. The kidney in gout. *Medicine.* 1960; 39:405–67.

729. Talbott JH, Yü TF. *Gout and Uric Acid Metabolism.* New York: Stratton Intercontinental Medical Book Corporation, 1976.

730. Tanquerel des Planches L. *Lead Diseases: A Treatise from the French of L Tanquerel des Planches with Notes and Additions on the Rise of Lead Pipe and its Substitutes.* Translated by SL Dana. Boston: Tappan, Whittemore & Mason, 1850.

731. Tara S, Françon F. Deux cas de goutte saturnine à modalité mineure. *Rhumatology.* 1957; 5:238–43.

732. Taussig CW. *Rum, Romance and Rebellion.* New York: Minton, Balch and Co, 1928.

733. Taylor AS. *On Poisons in Relation to Medical Jurisprudence.* Philadelphia: Lea and Blanchard, 1848.

734. ———. *Medical Jurisprudence and Medicine.* 3rd ed. Philadelphia: Henry C Lea, 1875.

735. Teisinger J, Srbova J. The value of mobilization of lead by calcium ethylene-diamine-tetra-acetate in the diagnosis of lead poisoning. *Brit J Indust Med.* 1959; 16:148–52.

736. Teleky L. *History of Factory and Mine Hygiene.* New York: Columbia Univ. Press, 1948.

737. Temple W. *An Essay upon the Cure of the Gout by Moxa.* London: AM and RR for Edw Gellibrand, 1680.

738. ———. *Miscellanea the Third Part.* London: Jonathan Swift, 1701.

739. Tepper EF, Lebanthal M, Haddad B, Sampson L, Wedeen RP. Does lead cause gout nephropathy? *Clin Res.* 1979; 27:500A.

740. Tepper L. Renal function subsequent to childhood plumbism. *Arch Environ Health.* 1963; 7:76–85.

741. Thacher J. *American Modern Practice, or, a Simple Method of Prevention and Cure of Diseases.* Boston: Ezra Read, 1817.

742. ———. *American Medical Biography.* Boston, 1828. Reprint, 1967.

743. Thackeray WM. *The Four Georges: Sketches of Manners, Morals, Court and Town Life.* London: Adam and Charles Black, 1910.

744. Thackrah CT. *The Effects of the Principal Arts, Trade and Professions, and of Civic States and Habits of Living, on Health and Longevity.* Philadelphia: L Johnson, 1831.

745. Theophilus. *On Divers Arts—The Foremost Medieval Treatise on Painting, Glassmaking and Metalwork.* Translated by JG Hawthorne and CS Smith. New York: Dover Publications, 1963/1979.

746. Theophrastus. *On Stones.* Translated by ER Caley and JFC Richards. Columbus: Ohio State Univ. 1956.

747. Thompson CJS. *The Quacks of London.* Philadelphia: JB Lippincott, 1929.

748. Tissot SAD. *Practical Observations on the Smallpox, the Apoplexy, Dropsy, and Nervous Cholic.* Dublin: James Williams, 1773.

749. Todd RB. *Practical Remarks on Gout, Rheumatic Fever, and Chronic Rheumatism of the Joints.* London: John W Parker, 1843.

750. ———. Clinical lecture on various cases. *Lond Med Gaz.* 1851; 48:1045–52.

751. ———. *Clinical Lectures on Certain Diseases of the Urinary Organs: and on Dropsies.* London: John Churchill, 1857.

752. Tronchin T. *A Treatise on the Colica Pictonum; or the Dry Belly-Ach.* Translated by R Schomberg. London: W Johnston, 1764.

753. Trotter T. *An Essay, Medical, Philosophical, and Chemical, on Drunkenness, and its Effects on the Human Body.* 2nd ed. London: Longmans, Hurst, Rees, Orme, 1804.

754. Turner AJ. On lead poisoning in childhood. *Br Med J.* 1909; 1:895–97.

755. USDHEW, NIOSH. *Criteria for a Recommended Standard—Occupational Exposure to Inorganic Lead.* 1972.

756. ———. *Criteria for a Recommended Standard—Occupational Exposure to Inorganic Lead. Revised Criteria.* 1978.

757. USDHEW, OSHA. Occupational exposure to lead final standard. *Federal Register.* Nov. 14, 1978: 52953–53014.

758. Urdang G. *Pharmacopeia Londinensis of 1618.* Hollister Pharmaceutical Library, Number 2. Madison: State Historical Society of Wisconsin, 1944.

759. Ursinus L. *Disputatio Medica Inauguralis de Morbis Metallariorum.* Leipzig: Bach, 1652.

760. Vangelista A, Caudarella R, Bonomini V. Lead poisoning nephropathy. *Abstracts: Int Congress Nephrol.* 1978; 7:D32.

761. Vaquez MH. La tension artérielle dans le saturnisme aigu et chronique. *Semin Med*. 1904; 48:385−87.

762. Vaugham WT. Lead poisoning from drinking "moonshine" whiskey. *JAMA*. 1922; 79:966.

763. Verger D, Leroux-Robert C, Ganther P, Richet G. Les tophus goutteux de la médullaire rénale des urémiques chroniques. *Nephron*. 1967; 4:356−70.

764. Vernatti P. A relation of the making of Ceruss. *Phil Tr Roy Soc, Lond*. 1678; 12:935−36.

765. Vicarius JJF. De vino lythargyriato. Unpublished translation by M. Sollenberger. *Miscellanea Curiosa sive Ephemeridum Medico-Physicarum Germanicarum*. 1st ed. 1691. 1697:208−14.

766. Vigdortchik NA. Lead intoxication in the etiology of hypertonia. *J Ind Hyg*. 1935; 17:1−6.

767. Virchow R. Seltene Gichtablagerungen. *Virchows Arch Path Anat*. 1868; 44:137−38.

768. Vitale LF, Joselow MM, Wedeen RP. Blood lead—an inadequate measure of occupational exposure. *J Occup Med*. 1975; 17:155−56.

769. Volhard F. Elevated blood-pressure. Chapter XXIII. In: Berglund H, ed. *The Kidney in Health and Disease*. Philadelphia: Lea and Febiger, 1935.

770. Wagner G. Evidence for third millenium lead-silver mining on Siphnos Island (Cyclades). *Naturwissenschaften*. 1979; 66:157−58.

771. Wai CM, Knowles CR, Keely JF. Lead caps on wine bottles and their potential problems. *Bull Environ Contam Toxicol*. 1979; 21:4−6.

772. Wainewright J. *A Mechanical Account of the Non-Naturals . . .* 5th ed. London: John Clarke, 1737.

773. Waldron HA. James Hardy and the Devonshire colic. *Med Hist*. 1969; 13:74−81.

774. ⸺. A note on the sensitivity of a method used to detect lead in the eighteenth century. *Br J Ind Med*. 1973; 30:300.

775. Waldron T. Did Hippocrates describe lead poisoning? *Lancet*. 1978; ii:1315.

776. Wall M. *Medical Tracts by the Late John Wall MD, of Worcester*. Oxford: D Prince, J Cooke, T Cadell, 1780.

777. Wallace SL. Colchicum: the panacea. *Bull NY Acad Med*. 1973; 49:130−35.

778. Wallace SL, Bernstein D. The relationship between gout and the kidney. *Metabolism*. 1963; 12:440−46.

779. Warner F. *A Full and Plain Account of the Gout*. 2nd ed. London: James Williams, 1769.

780. Waterhouse B. *Cautions to Young Persons Concerning Health . . .* Cambridge: At the University Press, 1805.

781. Watson CJ, Larson EA. The urinary coproporphyrins in health and disease. *Phys Rev*. 1947; 27:478−510.

782. Watson CJ, Schwartz S. A simple test for urinary porphobilinogen. *Proc Soc Exp Biol Med*. 1941; 47:393−94.

783. Webb W. *An Inaugural Dissertation on the Colic*. Philadelphia: John Ormrod, 1798.

784. ———. The lead-miners of Derbyshire: and their diseases. *Brit Med J.* 1857; 33:685–88.

785. Webster J. *Metallographia or an History of Metals.* Facsimile. New York: Arno Press, 1978.

786. Wedeen RP. Lead nephropathy. *Am J Med.* 1976; 61:583–84.

787. ———. Hyperuricemia and gouty nephropathy: the persisting controversy. *Drug Therapy.* 1981; 11:45–52.

788. ———. "Punch Cures the Gout." *J Med Soc NJ.* 1981; 78:201–6.

789. ———. Lead nephrotoxicity. In: Porter G, ed. *Nephrotoxic Mechanisms of Drugs and Environmental Toxins.* New York: Plenum Pub Co, 1982.

790. ———. The role of lead in renal failure. *Clin Exp Dialysis Apheresis.* 1982; 6:113–46.

791. ———. Occupational renal disease. *Am J Kid Disease.* 1984; 3:241–57.

792. Wedeen RP, Batuman V, Landy E. The safety of the EDTA lead-mobilization test. *Environ Res.* 1983; 30:58–62.

793. Wedeen RP, Maesaka JK, Weiner B, Lipat GA, Lyons MM, Vitale LF, Joselow NM. Occupational lead nephropathy. *Am J Med.* 1975; 59:630–41.

794. Wedeen RP, Mallik DK, Batuman V. Detection and treatment of occupational lead nephropathy. *Arch Intern Med.* 1979; 139:53–57.

795. Wedeen RP, Mallik DF, Batuman V, Bogden JD. Geographic lead nephropathy: a case report. *Environ Res.* 1978; 17:409–15.

796. Weinman EJ. Uric acid and the kidney. *Perspectives in Hypertension.* 1976; 3:141–58.

797. Weiss S, Parker F. Pyelonephritis: its relation to vascular lesions and to arterial hypertension. *Medicine.* 1939; 18:221–315.

798. Wells WC. On the presence of the red matter and serum of blood in the urine of dropsy, which has not originated from scarlet fever. *Tr Soc Improve Med Chir Knowl.* 1812; 3:194–240.

799. Wepfer JJ. Paresis post colicum ex vino. Unpublished translation by M. Sollenberger. *Micellanea Curiosa, sive Ephemeridum Medico-Physicarum Germanicarum Curiosarum, Annus Secundus, Anni scilicet DCLXXI.* Frankfurt, 1688:70–71.

800. Wertime TA. Man's first encounters with metallurgy. *Science.* 1964; 146:1257–67.

801. Wesley J. *Primitive Physic: or, an Easy and Natural Method for Curing most Diseases.* 16th ed. London: R Hawes, 1774.

802. ———. *Primitive Physic: or, an Easy and Natural Method of Curing Most Diseases. To Which is Added the General Receipt Both Containing Upwards Four Hundred of the Valuable Receipts.* London, 1845.

803. Westerman MP, Pfitzer E, Ellis LD, Jensen WN. Concentrations of lead in bone in plumbism. *N Engl J Med.* 1965; 273:1246–50.

804. Westfall RS. *Never at Rest: A Biography of Isaac Newton.* Cambridge: Cambridge Univ. Press, 1980.

805. Whitaker JA, Austin W, Nelson JD. Edathamil calcium disodium (Versenate) diagnostic test for lead poisoning. *Pediatrics.* 1962; 29:384–88.

806. Wickham E. Observation d'intoxication saturnine. Névropathie. Albuminurie. Guérison. *L'Union Med.* 1888; 45:969–76.

807. Wilks S. Saturnine gout. *Br Med J.* 1875; 1:9–10.

808. Willes RF, Truelove JF. Retention and tissue distribution of ^{210}Pb $(NO_3)_2$ administered orally to infant and adult monkeys. *J Toxicol Environ Health.* 1977; 3:395–406.

809. Williams B. Gout. *Med J Aust.* 1975; 1:368.

810. Wills G. *The Book of Copper and Brass.* London: Hamilton Pub Group, 1968.

811. Wilson JD, Simmonds HA, North JDK. Allopurinol in the treatment of uraemic patients with gout. *Ann Rheum Dis.* 1967; 26:136–42.

812. Wilson M. De la colique à laquelle sont exposés les ouvriers qui travaillent aux mines de plomb de Lead-Hils, extraite d'une lettre écute. *J de med chir et pharmacie.* 1758; 8:133–36.

813. Wilson VK, Thomson ML, Dent CE. Aminoaciduria in lead poisoning. *Lancet.* 1953; ii:66–68.

814. Wirtzung C. *Praxis medicinae Universalis . . .* Translated by IM Germane. London: George Bishop, 1598.

815. Withering W. *An Account of the Fox Glove . . .* Birmingham: S Swinney, 1785.

816. Wollaston WH. On gouty and urinary concretions. *Philo Tr Roy Soc, Lond.* 1797; 87:386–400.

817. Woodall J. *The Surgeons Mate.* London: R Young, 1639.

818. Wooliscroft JO, Colfer H, Fox IH. Hyperuricemia in acute illness: a poor prognostic sign. *Am J Med.* 1982; 72:58–62.

819. World Health Organization (WHO). *Environmental Health Criteria 3. Lead.* Geneva: World Health Organization, 1977.

820. Wright T, Evans RH. *Account of the Caricatures of James Gillray.* New York: B Blom, 1968.

821. Wyngaarden JB. The role of the kidney in the pathgenesis and treatment of gout. *Arthritis Rheum.* 1958; 1:191–203.

822. Wyngaarden JB, Kelley Wn. *Gout and Hypeuricaemia.* New York: Grune and Stratton, 1976.

823. Yü TF, Berger L. Impaired renal function in gout: its association with hypertensive vascular disease and intrinsic renal disease. *Am J Med.* 1982; 72:95–100.

824. Yü TF, Berger L, eds. *The Kidney in Gout and Hyperuricemia.* Mt Kisco, NY: Futura Pub Co, 1982.

825. Yü TF, Berger L, Dorph DJ, Smith H. Renal function in gout. V. Factors influencing the renal hemodynamics. *Am J Med.* 1979; 67:766–71.

826. Zimmer FE. Lead poisoning in scrap-metal workers. *JAMA.* 1961; 175:238–40.

Addenda

A1. Benedek TG. The gout of Desiderius Erasmus and Willibald Pirckheimer: medical, autobiography and its literary reflections. *Bull Hist Med*. 1984; 57:526–44.
A2. Drake R. *An Essay on the Nature and Manner of Treating the Gout*. London: Drake, 1758.
A3. Oliver T. A clinical lecture on lead-poisoning. *Brit Med J*. 1885; 2:731–35.

Index

105; emetics, 136; garlic, 23; horseback riding, 83; lead, 18, 55, 57,
108, 109; urine, 108; venesection,
93, 114; water, 121, 122. *See also*
Bath; Colchicine; Moxa; Wine,
medicinal
Gout, irregular: in birds, 200; symptoms, 83, 97, 105–9, 135; terminology, 80, 97, 106–8, 112, 188,
191, 214. *See also* Colic; Nephropathy; Palsy; Porphyria; Rum; Wine
Gout, saturnine, 18, 21, 82, 129; colic
of Poitou, 20; controversy, 39, 40;
Devonshire colic, 26; in England,
108, 133–35, 138, 189; in France,
161–63, 193–96, 204; in Germany,
21, 204; overlooked, 129, 160, 212,
213; in the United States, 116, 170,
180, 214; uric acid, 189, 190. *See
also* Anemia; Glazes; Hardy, James;
Lead workers; Nephropathy, lead;
Wepfer, Johann Jacob
Gouty kidney. *See* Nephropathy, gout
Goyer, Robert, 170
Graham, William, 174
Grant, William, 136
Greece: gout, 76; lead mines, 11; medicinal lead, 51; silver, 13; wine, 40;
uroscopy, 143
Grew, Nehemiah, 56
Gripes, 40–50. *See also* Bellyache,
dry; Gout of the stomach

Haen, Anton de, 32, 56, 58, 193
Haig, Alexander, 116
Hamilton, Alice, 72, 180
Hamilton, James, 156
Hardy, James, 39, 40, 131–34
Harlan, Richard, 60
Harrington, John, 16, 78
Harrison, James Bowen, 160
Harvey, William, 83
Heart disease: enlarged, 208, 209;
lead, 172; proteinuria, 161, 195. *See
also* Dropsy
Heberden, William, 134, 135
Hellebore. *See* Colchicine

Hematuria (blood in urine), 142, 212
Heme. *See* Anemia
Hemodactyl. *See* Colchicine
Henderson, D. A., 166
High blood pressure. *See* Hypertension
Hill, John, 56, 119
Hillary, William, 41, 47, 49, 114
Hippocrates, 54, 126; colic, 40; gout,
76, 80, 184, 190; hemorrhage, 51;
kidney disease, 143; lead, 13. *See
also* Paracelsians
Hoffman, Frederick, 184
Hooke, Robert, 56, 147
Humors, 15, 18, 20, 21, 54, 55, 106,
108, 136
Hunt, J., 121
Husson, 105, 125
Hüttenkatz, 21
Huxham, John, 26, 31, 32, 38, 48, 56,
133, 134
Hydrochloric acid (muriatic acid),
125, 186, 188
Hydrogen sulfide, 30
Hypertension: essential, 209–11;
gout, 204, 208, 210, 213; from kid-
ney disease, 207, 210, 211; from
lead, 169, 172, 192, 210; porphyria,
88
Hyperuricemia. *See* Uric acid

Immunology: and hypertension, 211
Industry, lead, 4, 16, 65–73, 218;
ILZRO (International Lead Zinc Re-
search Organization), 173
Infection, urinary tract, 207. *See also*
Pyelonephritis
Ingram, Dale, 184
Insanity. *See* Encephalopathy
Interstitial nephritis. *See* Nephritis,
interstitial
Iron therapy, 65
Islam. *See* Arabian medicine

James, Robert, 23, 56, 70
Jersey City, 4
John XXI (Pope), 76
Johnson, Samuel, 82

Richard P. Wedeen, M.D., F.A.C.P., is

Associate Chief of Staff for

Research and Development,

Veterans Administration Medical Center,

East Orange, New Jersey, and

Professor of Medicine,

University of Medicine and Dentistry of New Jersey,

New Jersey Medical School, Newark.